Maximize Your Health

The Top Ten Research Proven Strategies To Reduce Your Risk Of Chronic Disease

Dr. Thomas L. Halton

Published by
Fitness Plus

First Edition

Published by Fitness Plus
Boston, MA

ISBN 978-0-9882314-0-5

Table of Contents

Disclaimer

This book is intended for informational and educational purposes only. It is not meant to provide counseling, nor to provide medical advice. Always be sure to consult with your physician before starting any exercise program.

Introduction

Enjoying life to the fullest extent. Feeling good physically and mentally as long as we possibly can. Isn't that the ultimate goal for all of us at the end of the day? Don't we all want to push off our inevitable meeting with the grim reaper for as long as possible? Speaking for myself, the answer is an overwhelming yes.

Many people feel that when their number is up, it is up. Their cause of death has been programmed into their genes from the time they were born. I strongly disagree. I've been studying the prevention of chronic disease and helping people to improve their health for well over 15 years, and I'm not afraid to say that I have learned quite a bit. After you finish reading this book, you will know what I know.

I strongly believe that how we live our lives today will dictate how and when we will die. We have a lot more control than most people think. Unfortunately, the majority of us aren't paying nearly enough attention to what we can change. It is my sincere goal in writing this book to help you change this situation. But first things first. As I always do with a new client, allow me to introduce myself.

About Me

My name is Dr. Thomas L. Halton. I am a recent graduate of Harvard University with a Doctorate in Nutritional Epidemiology. What exactly does that mean? Well, epidemiology is simply the study of disease. So, my degree has taught me all about how nutrition impacts risk of disease, both positively and negatively. My main focus was heart disease, diabetes, stroke, cancer, and obesity. I also hold Masters Degrees in Exercise Science and Human Nutrition. I am a Certified Nutrition Specialist, a Licensed Dietician in the state of Massachusetts, and a Certified Personal Trainer by the American Council on Exercise.

I do have a great deal of academic experience, but I have an even greater amount of clinical experience. I founded and run Fitness Plus, a nutrition counseling and personal training company based in Boston, MA. For over 15 years, I've been helping people improve their lives with the right combination of nutrition and exercise.

A lot of my clients need to lose weight, but others have an increased risk of heart disease, type 2 diabetes, stroke, and cancer. They work with me to help them reduce this risk. I even have a group of doctors in the Boston area that send me out to see each of their patients to teach them what I know about how diet and exercise can improve their health.

My academic background has taught me a ton of research on how diet, exercise, and our lifestyle can increase or decrease risk of disease. My clinical experience has taught me how to help people apply the principles that I have learned in the real and busy world of job and family responsibilities.

I wrote this book because I have yet to see a simple, easy to read and research based manual on what we need to be doing to reduce our risk of chronic disease. My goal is not only to emphasize the important factors, but also explain why they are important from a research perspective. One thing I've learned about almost any problem in life is that half of the solution lies in knowing what is wrong. The desire and ability to change these factors will vary considerably from reader to reader, but you will have the knowledge of what to do after reading this book.

I'm astounded by the conflicting health information that confuses the public in the fields of exercise and nutrition. There is a huge and wonderful body of scientific research literature that sheds light on how diet and exercise can improve our health. Yet most people, including many doctors, are completely unaware of it. It is my hope that this book will summarize what we currently know in these fields and help you understand what factors are the most important for you to focus upon. It is also my goal to keep the tone of the book agreeable for those who have not studied research methodology.

Causes Of Death In The U.S.

Before we jump into how we'll prevent disease, it is important to know which diseases are the most common. According to the latest statistics from the Centers for Disease Control, the top cause of death in the U.S. is heart disease, which claims roughly 600,000 lives each year. A close second is cancer at 567,628 deaths per year. The number three cause of death is chronic respiratory disease at 137,353 deaths per year. The fourth leading cause of death is stroke at 128,842 deaths per year (1).

A closer examination shows that for cancer, the top three causes of cancer death account for just about two-thirds of all cancer deaths. For men, it is lung cancer, prostate cancer, and then colon cancer. For women, it is lung cancer, breast cancer, and then colon cancer (2). As you read the rest of this book, keep these stats in mind. These are the diseases that are the most likely to affect you and the ones you should most focus on preventing. The good news is that your odds of developing these diseases are highly modifiable.

Top 4 Causes of Death In the U.S.
#1 Heart Disease 599,413
#2 Cancer 567,628
#3 Respiratory Disease 137,353
#4 Stroke 128,842

Source: Center For Disease Control (Reference 1)

Research 101

It is important to understand just the tiniest bit of research design in order to properly interpret the literature that will be referred to in this book. I promise to keep this as short and painless as possible. Although there are five different types of study design (ecological, cross-sectional, case-control, cohort, and experimental), the two that will be the most relevant for us are the cohort study and the experimental study.

Experimental Studies

Experimental studies are also known as intervention studies, trials, or clinical trials. Whatever you call them, they are the absolute gold standard of research design. If conducted correctly, they are the design that will give you the very best chance of answering your research question with confidence.

In clinical trials, an exposure is tested to see if it causes, prevents, or treats a disease. The researcher will take a population, split it in half and give one group the exposure variable while the other group gets a placebo. After a period of time, you compare rates of disease between the two groups.

Example: Vitamin C And The Common Cold

Here's an example of a clinical trial. Say you want to see if vitamin C supplements can prevent the common cold. You have 100 study participants in this intervention. First you would randomly split them into two groups of 50.

The first group is called the intervention group. This group will receive 1,000 mg. of vitamin C in pill form each day from September 1st through March 31st (cold season). The second group of 50 does not get the vitamin C. They get a pill called a placebo that looks just like the vitamin C pill but has no active ingredients. This is done so the participants and even most of the researchers won't really know who is getting the vitamin C and who is not. This way, the results reported will be more objective.

During the follow-up period of September 1st to March 31st, the number of colds in each group is recorded, added up, and compared. In our fictional study, the vitamin C group had a total of 35 colds while the placebo group had 34 colds. You can then analyze these numbers to see if they are statistically different. In this case, both groups got sick just about the same number of times, so it doesn't look like vitamin C had a preventative effect.

So, why are clinical trials considered the gold standard of research? It all has to do with the traits of the intervention group compared to the placebo group. If your assignment of subjects to the groups is truly

objective and random, the groups are identical in every way except for the fact that one gets the exposure you are testing and the other does not.

So in our fictional study, the two groups would be similar in age, weight, physical activity, smoking habits, and any other number of factors. In fact, the only real difference between the two groups is that one received the vitamin C pill and the other a placebo. This way you can really learn if vitamin C affected the rate of illness because everything else about the groups is the same. If your study sample is large enough and your groups are similar enough, you are truly isolating the effects of the vitamin C on the common cold. Every other factor that may impact the odds of coming down with a cold is the same in both groups.

Although the trial is considered the best way to examine a research question, there are definitely times when a trial is not feasible:

1) Trials are extremely expensive. Sometimes a budget simply won't allow for a randomized trial.
2) Some diseases take 10, 20, or even 30 years to develop. Cancer, atherosclerosis, heart disease, stroke, and type 2 diabetes are examples of diseases that can take decades to progress. It is not realistic to keep people enrolled in a trial for 10 or 20 years.
3) Ethical issues can prevent the use of the trial design. For example, it has been theorized for years that smoking causes lung cancer. It would

> not be ethical to put a group of subjects in a smoking intervention to see if smoking indeed causes lung cancer. If you're right, you've killed a bunch of innocent people. Not good!!!

For occasions such as these, the next best bet is the cohort study.

Cohort Studies

A cohort is simply a group of individuals that share an experience or characteristic trait. For example, all females that are registered nurses in the United States would be a cohort. Everyone who lives in Framingham, MA is another example of a cohort. A cohort is just a bunch of people that have something in common.

In a cohort study, a group of individuals with a variety of exposures are studied for a length of time to determine the occurrence of disease or death. This is an example of observational research. The researchers just watch, they don't tell anyone to do anything. This helps to avoid the ethical dilemmas that often pop up when conducting trials.

The idea is that if your cohort is large enough, just by the law of averages, you will have variety in exposures. For example, if you went to your local shopping mall and randomly picked 100 people and had them fill out a questionnaire, chances are that some of them would smoke and some would not. Some would be thin and others would be overweight. Some would eat a healthy diet and some would eat terribly.

Now multiply that 100 people to 1,000 people, or 10,000 people or even 100,000. When you get a group that size, you will have variety in just about every exposure imaginable. These studies offer almost limitless opportunity to study all sorts of diseases and all sorts of causes of those diseases. While I was at Harvard, I was privileged to work on two of the absolute best cohort studies in the entire world: The Nurses' Health Study and The Health Professionals Study.

The Nurses' Health Study

The Nurses' Health Study is an example of an amazing cohort study that was initiated in 1976 and continues today. In 1976, 121,700 U.S. female registered nurses were identified and asked to provide comprehensive information about their health and lifestyle (3).

They were asked about their age, weight, height, smoking habits, exercise habits, if they had been diagnosed with any diseases or conditions, if they take medication, and a bunch of other questions. Every two years, questionnaires were sent out to all participants to update these lifestyle factors and inquire about new disease diagnoses.

In 1980, a 131 item food frequency questionnaire was mailed out in order to assess the participant's diet. This food frequency questionnaire is a remarkable tool developed by the head of the Harvard University Department of Nutrition, Dr. Walter Willett. This questionnaire changed the way we conduct nutrition research forever because it has the ability to accurately measure diet over the previous year.

Earlier methods of assessing diet, such as the 24 hour dietary recall or the one week diet record, didn't really reflect usual intake and were more of a snap shot of a person's diet. The food frequency questionnaire has been sent out every four years since 1980 to update changes in the nurses' diet over time.

With all of this information, researchers can conduct an almost limitless variety of research investigations. For example, you can divide the women into high or low consumption of trans fat and then wait to see who develops heart disease and who doesn't. You can look at almost any dietary variable and almost any medical outcome. Since the Nurses' Health Study began over 35 years ago, a ton of great research has been published.

A similar cohort study at Harvard is the Health Professional Follow-up Study, which was initiated in 1986 and consists of 51,529 males in the health field (dentists, pharmacists, optometrists, etc). Like the Nurses' Health Study, the Health Professional Follow-up Study continues to this very day.

I conducted much of my research while at Harvard on the Nurses' Health Study and also ran some analyses on the Health Professional Follow-up Study. Throughout the remainder of this book, I will reference studies from these two cohorts as well as other cohort studies and clinical trials to help give teeth to my lifestyle recommendations.

Book Layout

The remainder of this book will consist of 10 short chapters that will, in order of importance, illustrate the most pertinent modifiable risk factors to maintain your health. Each lifestyle factor will be explained, a synopsis of the current research will be presented, and then a take home recommendation will be offered.

If you are able to follow these 10 recommendations, I am quite convinced that you will dramatically reduce your risk of today's most deadly killers, including heart disease, stroke, cancer, and diabetes. Some of these factors will be nutritional in nature, others will be more lifestyle oriented. All will be backed by the latest research at the time of this writing. For the academic types among you, I will provide references for further reading.

There is a lot of information out there telling us how to live in order to promote health and reduce risk of disease. Much of it is conflicting. It is my goal in writing this book to shed some light on the really important factors and separate opinion from research based hypothesis.

Let's get started!!!

TAKE HOME MESSAGE

1) The top four causes of death in the U.S. are: heart disease, cancer, respiratory disease, and stroke.
2) The risk for these diseases is highly modifiable. The way you live your life has much to do with your chances of developing these diseases.
3) Following are the 10 most important things you can do, in order of importance, to stay healthy. The more of these you follow, the lower your risk of disease and early mortality.

References

1) http://www.cdc.gov/nchs/fastats/lcod.htm

2) http://apps.nccd.cdc.gov/uscs/toptencancers.aspx

3) Stampfer MJ, Hu FB, Manson JE, et al. Primary prevention of coronary heart disease in women through diet and lifestyle. *New England Journal of Medicine* 2000; 343:16-22.

Priority #1
Don't Smoke

This one should not come as a surprise to any of you. Avoiding smoking gets the nod for the #1 way to reduce your risk of deadly disease. It wasn't even close. Most of us know how bad smoking is for our health. We are told at a young age not to do it. To be honest, I never really knew just how bad it was until I started studying epidemiology. I think you'll be a bit surprised by some of the facts that you'll read in this chapter.

What Is In Cigarettes, Anyway?

There are 4,000 distinct chemicals in cigarette smoke. Two hundred and fifty are known to be harmful to humans, including hydrogen cyanide, carbon monoxide, and ammonia (1). Sixty-nine of these are known to cause cancer, including arsenic, benzene, and formaldehyde (1). At the time of this writing, 20.6% of U.S. adults smoke cigarettes and fully 20% of U.S. high school students smoke (2). These numbers are down from decades ago but they are still far too high.

Cost Of Smoking In The United States

Smoking is considered the single greatest cause of avoidable morbidity and mortality in the United States. It is responsible for approximately 440,000 deaths each year (3). Of this number, 40% are from cancer, 35% from heart disease, and 25% from lung disease (1). Each year, smoking results in $157 billion in annual health related economic losses and 5.6 million years of potential life lost (3). This is no joke people! If you desire to live a long and healthy life and you are currently smoking, it is time to wake up! A great doctor I know calls smoking, "Suicide on the installment plan".

Here is a list of diseases that have been associated with cigarette smoking:

Diseases Associated With Smoking

Bladder Cancer	Cervical Cancer
Esophageal Cancer	Kidney Cancer
Laryngeal Cancer	Leukemia
Lung Cancer	Oral Cancer
Pancreatic Cancer	Stomach Cancer
Abdominal Aortic Aneurysm	Stroke
Atherosclerosis	Peptic Ulcer
Coronary Heart Disease	Pneumonia
Chronic Obstructive Pulmonary Disease	Low Birth Weight
	Cataracts
Decreased Fertility	Hip Fracture

Source: Reference #3

Second Hand Smoke

When you smoke, you not only severely undermine your own health, but you also damage anyone whose lungs are in range of your toxic exhalation—including your spouse and children. It is estimated that annually in the U.S., 49,400 deaths are caused by the effects of second hand smoke (2). Among these are 3,000 lung cancer deaths and 46,000 deaths from coronary heart disease (1). The Surgeon General estimates that living with a smoker increases a non-smoker's risk of lung cancer by 20-30% and heart disease by 25-30% (4). In fact, second hand smoke is now classified as a known carcinogen by the United States National Toxicology Program (5).

Smoking In The Nurses' Health Study

As I mentioned in the first chapter, the Nurses' Health Study is a cohort study that I worked on while I was at Harvard. A number of papers have been published that have examined the effects of smoking on the health of women in this cohort.

Smoking And Lung Cancer In The Nurses' Health Study

In 2008, researchers from Harvard published a comprehensive paper on the effects of smoking in women from the Nurses' Health Study (6). The study followed 104,519 women for 24 years (from 1980-2004). During that time there were 12,483 deaths.

Following are the risks of lung cancer for smokers in comparison to those that never smoked:

Women smoking 1-14 cigarettes per day had 12 times the risk of lung cancer when compared to never smokers.

Women smoking 15-24 cigarettes per day had approximately 23 times the risk of lung cancer when compared to never smokers.

Women smoking 25-34 cigarettes per day had approximately 30 times the risk of lung cancer when compared to never smokers.

Women smoking greater than 35 cigarettes per day had approximately 40 times the risk of lung cancer when compared to never smokers.

The risk of lung cancer for quitters approached the level of non-smokers after 30 years.

As mentioned earlier, cigarettes contain a large number of toxic compounds that are directly carcinogenic to lung tissue.

Risk Of Heart Attack

In 1987, Harvard researchers published a study in the *New England Journal of Medicine* detailing the effects of smoking on risk of coronary heart disease in women from the Nurses' Health Study. Over 119,400 women were followed for six years (7). Following are the major findings of this important investigation:

Women smoking 25 or more cigarettes per day had 5½ times the risk of fatal coronary heart disease when compared to never smokers.

Women smoking 25 or more cigarettes per day had 6 times the risk of non-fatal myocardial infarction when compared to never smokers.

Smoking 1-4 or 5-14 cigarettes each day was associated with a two to three fold increased risk of fatal coronary heart disease or non-fatal myocardial infarction.

In this cohort of female nurses, cigarette smoking accounted for 50% of all coronary heart disease events.

Former smokers had little if any of the risk.

Stroke

In 1988, Harvard researchers published a study in *The New England Journal of Medicine* that looked at the effects of smoking on risk of stroke in women in the Nurses' Health Study (8). Over 118,500 women were followed for eight years, and during this time there were 274 new cases of stroke.

Women who smoked 1-14 cigarettes per day had 2.2 times the risk of stroke compared to never smokers.

Women who smoked 25 cigarettes per day had 3.7 times the risk of never smokers.

Type 2 Diabetes

In 1993, Harvard published a study that examined the association between smoking and risk of type 2 diabetes in the Nurses' Health Study (9). This study was published in *The American Journal of Public Health*. Over 114,200 women were followed for 12 years, during which time there were 2,333 new cases of type 2 diabetes.

Women who smoked 25 or more cigarettes per day had a 42% increased risk of type 2 diabetes when compared to never smokers. The researchers theorized that smoking was directly toxic to pancreatic tissue (which produces insulin) and/or that smoking had a negative influence on waist to hip ratio. Both of these mechanisms potentially explain the increased risk of diabetes among smokers in this cohort.

Total Mortality

In a study mentioned in the earlier section on smoking and lung cancer, Harvard also looked at the effects of smoking on all causes of death over 22 years in 104,519 women in the Nurses' Health Study (6).

Women smoking 1-14 cigarettes per day had over 2 times the risk of dying from any cause compared to never smokers.

Women smoking 15-24 cigarettes per day had almost 3 times the risk of dying from any cause compared to never smokers.

Women smoking 25-34 cigarettes per day had 3½ times the risk.

Women smoking 35 or more cigarettes per day had 4 times the risk.

Recommendation For Smoking

The recommendations for smoking are quite simple. If you don't smoke, don't start. If you do smoke, you need to quit. You need to quit today. I've never smoked but I know that it is extremely addictive. There are a variety of programs available to aid you in ending your addiction to cigarettes. Some people find nicotine patches or gum effective. Others quit with the help of counseling or hypnosis. Others find support groups effective. Many can quit on their own.

It doesn't really matter how you do it, it is just imperative that you do it. This is the single most important thing you can do to preserve your health. Smoking is akin to playing Russian roulette with your risk of chronic disease. If staying healthy isn't important enough for you to give up cigarettes for good, then consider the following:

*You are hurting the people around you with your second hand smoke. This includes your kids and your spouse.

*Cigarettes cost a lot of money.

*Cigarettes make your breath, hair, and clothes smell terrible.

*Children often replicate their parents' health habits. Do you really want your kids to grow up thinking it's OK to smoke?

If you need some help quitting smoking, check out the American Lung Association website www.lungusa .org for more information.

TAKE HOME MESSAGE

1) Smoking cigarettes is the single worst thing that you can do for your health.
2) If you don't currently smoke, don't start!
3) If you do smoke, quit right away. I know that it's hard to quit, but it's also hard to deal with lung cancer, heart disease, and stroke at a young age. Where there is a will, there is a way. There are a variety of programs to help you with this. Ask your doctor and keep trying them until one works!
4) No matter how long you've smoked, there are both immediate and long term benefits to quitting.

References

1) http://www.cancer.gov/cancertopics/factsheet/tobacco/cessation

2) http://www.cancer.gov/cancertopics/tobacco/smoking

3) The Health Consequences of Smoking: A Report of the Surgeon General. Office of the Surgeon General (US); Office on Smoking and Health (US). Atlanta (GA): Centers for Disease Control and Prevention (US); 2004.

4) U.S. Department of Health and Human Services. *The Health Consequences of Involuntary Exposure to Tobacco Smoke: A Report of the Surgeon General.* Rockville, MD: U.S. Department of Health and Human Services, Centers for Disease Control and Prevention, Coordinating Center for Health Promotion, National Center for Chronic Disease Prevention and Health Promotion, Office on Smoking and Health, 2006.

5) National Toxicology Program. *Report on Carcinogens. Eleventh Edition.* U.S. Department of Health and Human Services, Public Health Service, National Toxicology Program, 2005.

6) Kenfield SA, Stampfer MJ, Rosner BA, et al. Smoking and smoking cessation in relation to mortality in women. *Journal of the American Medical Association* 2008; 299:2037-47.

7) Willett WC, Green A, Stampfer MJ, et al. Relative and absolute excess risks of coronary heart disease among women who smoke cigarettes. *New England Journal of Medicine* 1987; 317:1303-9.

8) Colditz GA, Bonita R, Stampfer MJ, et al. Cigarette smoking and risk of stroke in middle aged women. *New England Journal of Medicine* 1988; 318:937-41.

9) Rimm EB, Manson JE, Stampfer MJ, et al. Cigarette smoking and the risk of diabetes in women. *American Journal of Public Health* 1993; 83: 211-14.

Priority #2: Maintain A Healthy Weight

The second most important thing you can do to improve your health is to maintain a healthy body weight. Being overweight is second only to smoking in its ability to increase your risk of chronic disease. Humans were designed to be lean and mean. When you are overweight, your health is adversely affected in a frightening number of ways. The more overweight you are, the more serious the risks become.

How Do You Know If You Are Overweight?

The most common gauge of adiposity is the body mass index or BMI. This measure divides your weight in kilograms by your height in meters squared. The number you get is your BMI. If your BMI is under 25, you are considered normal weight. If you fall between 25-29.9, you are overweight, and if your number is 30 or more, you are considered obese. To find out your BMI, the Center for Disease Control has a free BMI calculator. Just go to www.cdc.gov and type "Body Mass Index" into the search box.

Another useful measure of how your weight is affecting your health is your waist circumference. Just take an old fashioned tape measure and loop it around your waist at your navel. If you are male, you want a waist below 40 inches. If you are female, you want a waist below 35 inches. Above these numbers, your risk of disease goes up sharply. Some older studies have also used waist to hip ratio, which is your waist divided by your hips. However, including the hips doesn't really add much predictive ability, so you can just stick with measuring your waist. Finally, one last useful measure used in a variety of studies is weight you have gained since the age of 18 years.

Prevalence And Economic Costs Of Obesity

According to The Center for Disease Control, one-third of U.S. adults are obese (more than 72 million) and 17% of our children are obese (1). When you add in those who are overweight (with a BMI between 25-29.9), fully two-thirds of Americans fall into the over-weight/obese category. It has gotten to the point that if you are at a healthy weight, you are in the minority in this country. What is truly scary about these numbers is how quickly they have climbed. Between 1980 and 2008, obesity rates for adults have doubled and for children they have tripled (1).

The economic burden of obesity is no less shocking. In 2008, obesity related costs were $147 billion, and an obese individual spends over $1,400 more in medical bills than someone with a normal weight (1). Following are some of the diseases that have been associated with overweight and obesity:

Diseases Associated With Overweight And Obesity

Heart Disease	Respiratory Disease
Stroke	Asthma
Hypertension	Early Death
High Cholesterol	Arthritis
Type 2 Diabetes	Infertility
Gall Bladder Disease	Sleep Apnea
A Variety Of Cancers	Cataracts

Now let's take a look at some of the important research on obesity and risk of disease.

All Cause Mortality

A number of large prospective studies have demonstrated that being overweight or obese increases the risk of dying from any cause.

The Nurses Health Study

In 1995, Harvard researchers published a study in *The New England Journal of Medicine* that looked at body mass index and risk of death from any cause in 115,195 women from the Nurses' Health Study (2). The women were followed for 16 years, and there were 4,726 deaths in the cohort during this time period. Compared to women with a BMI under 19, risk of dying was 30% higher for women with a BMI between 25-26.9, 60% higher for those with a BMI between 27-28.9, and over 2 times higher for women with a BMI over 29. The researchers noted that BMI was more strongly related to heart disease death than deaths from any other cause.

In 2008, Harvard researchers published a study in the journal *Circulation* that looked at waist circumference and risk of mortality in the Nurses' Health Study (3). The investigation included 44,636 nurses that were followed for 16 years. By the end of follow-up, there were 3,507 deaths (including 751 from cardiovascular disease and 1,748 from cancer). When comparing women with a waist circumference ≥35 to women with a waist circumference <28, there was a 71% increased risk of dying from any cause for the heavier women.

What was also interesting about this study was that even normal weight women (with a BMI less than 25) had an increased risk of dying if their waist circumference put them in the abdominally obese category (greater than 35 inches). The researchers assumed that the metabolic effects of abdominal obesity were responsible for the results, including insulin resistance, high cholesterol, and inflammation. These factors play a role in the incidence of cardiovascular disease, diabetes, and certain cancers.

Several other studies have confirmed the association between obesity and increased mortality. In the American Heart Association Cancer Prevention Study II cohort, which includes over 1 million subjects, men and women with the highest BMI had twice the risk of death compared to normal weight subjects over 14 years of follow-up (4). In the National Institutes of Health-AARP cohort, which includes over 500,000 subjects, BMI was linearly associated with mortality, with more than double the risk of death in the heaviest subjects (5). Finally, in the Shanghai Women's Health Study, 72,773 women were followed for an average of 5.7 years and women with the highest waist to hip ratio had approximately double the risk of dying from any cause compared to women with the lowest waist to hip ratio (6).

Coronary Heart Disease

Overweight and obesity have also been strongly associated with an increased risk of heart disease.

The Health Professional Follow-Up Study

In 1995, Harvard researchers published a study examining the association between weight and coronary heart disease in 29,122 men from the Health Professional Follow-up Study (7). In three years of follow-up, there were 420 cases of heart disease (which included fatal coronary heart disease, non-fatal myocardial infarction, bypass surgery or angioplasty). The analysis was focused on men under the age of 65.

When compared to men with a BMI less than 23, men with a BMI between 25-28.9 had a 70% increased risk of heart disease. Men with a BMI between 29-32.9 had a 2½ times increased risk of heart disease, and men with a BMI ≥33 had 3½ times the risk.

The Nurses Health Study

A similar analysis was also conducted in women from the Nurses' Health Study (8). Over 115,000 women were followed for 14 years. During this time, there were 1,292 new cases of heart disease (which included fatal heart disease or non-fatal myocardial infarction). Compared to women with a BMI less than 21, women with a BMI between 25-28.9 had more than double the risk of heart disease. Women with a BMI over 29 had a 3½ times increased risk of heart disease. Gaining weight after age 18 was also strongly associated with risk of heart disease. Even a modest gain of 11 pounds was associated with a 25% increased risk.

Excess weight increases the incidence of hypertension, insulin resistance, inflammation, and has a negative impact on serum cholesterol and triglyceride levels. These are all potential mechanisms by which being overweight increases the risk of coronary heart disease.

Cancer

American Cancer Society Cohort

The American Cancer Society published a study investigating the association between overweight and cancer in 750,000 men and women (9). After 12 years of follow-up, obese men had a 33% increased risk of cancer, while obese women had a 55% increased risk of cancer. For men, the risk was highest for colon and prostate cancer. For women, risk was highest for cancer of the endometrium, ovary, cervix, gallbladder, and breast.

The Nurses' Health Study

Researchers from Harvard also published a study on adult weight gain and risk of breast cancer in the Nurses' Health Study (10). Over 87,000 postmenopausal women were followed for up to 26 years. During this period there were 4,393 new cases of breast cancer. In a subset of the study, the researchers looked only at women who had never taken hormone replacement therapy. Among these women, risk of breast cancer increased 34% for those who gained between 22-44 pounds since age 18. Risk increased 55% for those gaining 44-55 pounds and doubled for women gaining more than 55 pounds since age 18.

The authors of the study theorized that the increased risk was due to endogenous hormone levels that increase with weight gain and may also increase the risk of breast cancer. Women who lost weight since age 18 had a decreased risk of breast cancer. Another interesting finding was that in those not taking post menopausal hormones, body weight accounted for 24% of all breast cancer in this cohort.

Type 2 Diabetes

The association between overweight and type 2 diabetes was examined in the Nurses' Health Study (11). Over 114,000 women were followed for 14 years, with 2,204 new cases of type 2 diabetes developing during that time. The results were striking. Compared to women with a BMI of less than 22, here are the risks of type 2 diabetes with increasing BMI:

Risk Of Type 2 Diabetes With Increasing BMI In The Nurses' Health Study

BMI	Risk Of Type 2 Diabetes
25-26.9	8 times increased risk
27-28.9	16 times increased risk
29-30.9	28 times increased risk
31-32.9	40 times increased risk
33-34.9	54 times increased risk
35+	93 times increased risk

The authors explained that the increased risk of diabetes with increasing BMI was most likely due to increased insulin resistance and deterioration of glucose tolerance.

Hypertension

The association between overweight and risk of hypertension was examined in the Nurses' Health Study (12). Over 82,000 women were followed for 16 years, and 16,395 new cases of hypertension were identified during that time. Compared to women with a

BMI under 20, women with a BMI between 25-25.9 had 2½ times the risk of developing hypertension. Women with a BMI between 26-27.9 had over 3 times the risk. Women with a BMI between 28-30.9 had 4 times the risk, and women with a BMI ≥31 had over 6 times the risk. The authors believed the increasing risk of hypertension with increasing BMI was due to an increased sympathetic nervous system activity, insulin resistance, high insulin levels, sodium retention, and /or enhanced vascular reactivity.

How To Maintain A Healthy Weight

I hope I've proven to you that being overweight is extremely damaging to your health. So what can one do to lose weight? As a Licensed Nutritionist, Exercise Physiologist, and Certified Personal Trainer, I have been helping people lose weight for over 15 years. I have developed a program that is both research based and extremely practical in the real world.

I have found that in order to lose weight and keep it off, three areas need attention. Here is the breakdown: 50% of your results will come from your diet, 30% of your results will come from your cardiovascular exercise, and 20% of your results will come from your resistance training program.

Diet

I have found that the most effective diet for weight loss is a low glycemic load, moderate fat regimen. With this style of eating, blood sugar becomes much more stable, resulting in a dramatic decrease in both hunger and food consumption.

There are two strategies to promote a stable blood sugar. The first strategy is to pick carbohydrate foods that will not cause a dramatic spike in blood sugar. These are known as low glycemic load carbohydrates. Examples include: fruits and vegetables, brown rice, oatmeal, and beans. It is also pivotal to limit high glyemic load carbohydrates; including bread, pasta, white rice, and sugar.

The second strategy to promote a stable blood sugar is to combine a source of healthy fat, lean protein, and low glyemic carbohydrate at each and every meal. The addition of fat and protein slows the entry of the carbohydrate into the blood stream. This will result in a more stable blood sugar, which is the key to weight loss.

Cardiovascular Exercise

Cardio is where you'll burn your calories and boost your metabolism. The research tells us that cardio has to be a daily occurrence if you are serious about losing weight and keeping it off. Most men will need to do 150 minutes of cardio each week to lose weight. Women have a slower metabolism and therefore have to work a little harder at their cardio. They generally will need to do 250 minutes of cardio each week in order to lose weight.

Resistance Training

Resistance training is the most overlooked aspect of weight loss programs. Once we hit our 25th birthday, we start to lose muscle at the rate of 1% each year. Since each pound of muscle burns roughly 50 calories per day, this is not good for our metabolism! Regular resistance training can not only stem this loss of muscle tissue, but can add to your lean body mass so that you will burn more calories each day.

You want to hit the weights at least twice per week and preferably three times per week. At a minimum, you'll want to do an exercise for your chest, back, shoulders, biceps, triceps, abs, and legs.

The details of these three components are beyond the scope of this chapter. In fact, there is so much more material to discuss on the subject, that I could fill a whole other book entirely. So, I figured I would go ahead and write that book! *The Weight Loss Triad*, by yours truly, lays out these three components in great detail. It is available on amazon.com. I truly believe this is a book that can change your life if you need to lose weight. (Sorry for the shameless plug!)

TAKE HOME MESSAGE

1) Humans were designed to be lean.
2) Overweight and obesity are associated with most major diseases, including: heart disease, stroke, diabetes, cancer, and early death.
3) Assess how your weight is impacting your health by learning your body mass index and waist circumference.
4) Maintain your weight by focusing on three areas: your diet, cardiovascular exercise, and resistance training.

References

1) http://www.cdc.gov/chronicdisease/resources/publications/AAG/obesity.htm

2) Manson JE, Willett WC, Stampfer MJ, et al. Body weight and mortality among women. *New England Journal of Medicine* 1995; 333:677-85.

3) Zhang C, Rexrode KM, Van Dam RM, et al. Abdominal obesity and the risk of all cause, cardiovascular, and cancer mortality: Sixteen years of follow up in U.S. women. *Circulation* 2008; 117:1658-1667.

4) Calle EE, Thun MT, Petrelli JM, et al. Body mass index and mortality in a prospective cohort of U.S. adults. *New England Journal of Medicine* 1999; 341: 1097-105.

5) Adams KF, Schatzkin A, Harris TB, et al. Overweight, obesity, and mortality in a large prospective cohort of persons 50-71 years old. *New England Journal of Medicine* 2006; 355: 763-78.

6) Zhang X, Shu XO, Yang G, et al. Abdominal adiposity and mortality in Chinese women. *Archives of Internal Medicine* 2007; 167:886-92.

7) Rimm EB, Stampfer MJ, Giovannucci E, et al. Body size and fat distribution as predictors of coronary heart disease among middle-aged and older U.S. men. *American Journal of Epidemiology* 1995; 141:1117-27.

8) Willett WC, Manson JE, Stampfer MJ, et al. Weight, weight change, and coronary heart disease in women. *Journal of the American Medical Association* 1995; 273:461-65.

9) Garfinkel L. Overweight and mortality. *Cancer* 1986; 58:1826-29.

10) Eliassen AH, Colditz GA, Rosner B, et al. Adult weight change and risk of postmenopausal breast cancer. *Journal of the American Medical Association* 2006; 296:193-201.

11) Colditz GA, Willett WC, Rotnitzky A, et al. Weight gain as a risk factor for clinical diabetes mellitus in women. *Annals of Internal Medicine* 1995; 122:481-486.

12) Huang Z, Willett WC, Manson JE, et al. Body weight, weight change and risk for hypertension in women. *Annals of Internal Medicine* 1998; 128:81-88.

Priority #3
Be Physically Active

Just imagine for a second if a new medication was introduced to the people of the United States that greatly enhanced weight loss. Imagine if the medication was also shown to reduce the risk of heart disease, stroke, diabetes, cancer, and Alzheimer's disease. This magical pill was also effective in reducing blood pressure, improving serum cholesterol, helped fight anxiety and depression, gave you more energy, boosted your immune system and mental focus, and even decreased your level of stress. Other side effects include improved sleep, more confidence, and an improved sex life.

It sounds too good to be true, right? If a drug like this ever came to market, I bet that over ¾ of U.S. adults would have a prescription for it inside of a month. Well, the above paragraph pretty much sums up the many benefits of being physically active. While there are a number of forms of physical activity, including weight training, flexibility training, and cardiovascular exercise, this chapter will largely focus on the benefits of cardiovascular exercise.

What Is Cardiovascular Exercise?

Cardiovascular exercise is any rhythmic, continuous movement of the large muscle groups that utilizes the aerobic system of energy production. Examples include: walking, jogging, elliptical training, stair climbing, rowing, cycling, and swimming. The human body was designed for movement, and we spent much of our early evolutionary period getting a ton of physical activity. I've read that our caveman ancestors walked 19 miles in a typical day!

Our bodies work best when we are active, and our systems start to break down when we are sedentary. As a country, we are not very active. Recently conducted surveys show that more than half of Americans do not attain the recommended levels of physical activity, and one in four reported absolutely no leisure time physical activity. This needs to change dramatically if we are to improve the health of this nation.

According to the latest *Physical Activity Guidelines for Americans*, the benefits of regular physical activity are numerous and continue to grow with new research (1). Following is a list of the diseases whose incidence decreases significantly with regular physical activity:

Physical Activity Reduces The Risk Of These Conditions And Diseases

Early Death	Heart Disease
Stroke	High Cholesterol
Type 2 Diabetes	Metabolic Syndrome
Colon Cancer	Breast Cancer
Obesity	Fall Prevention
Depression	Cognitive Dysfunction
Hip Fracture	Lung Cancer
Endometrial Cancer	Weight Regain
Osteoporosis	Insomnia

Source: 2008 Physical Activity Guidelines For Americans (1).

Look at that list again. It's hard to come up with a disease process that is not positively affected by physical activity. Let's take a quick look at the research from some of these major conditions, and then we'll get into some tips for building your own personal physical fitness program.

Total Mortality

The association between physical activity and death from all causes has been examined in a variety of studies over the years. We will briefly take a look at two of the larger and more influential investigations: The Cooper Aerobics Center Longitudinal Study and The Nurses' Health Study.

The Cooper Aerobics Center Longitudinal Study

The Cooper Longitudinal Study cohort is special because researchers measure actual cardio-respiratory fitness for each subject by means of a maximum treadmill test. Most of the other studies use questionnaires or self reported means of measuring physical activity. I've done some research consulting for The Cooper Institute located in Dallas, Texas, and let me say it's a pretty impressive place with some pretty impressive research capabilities.

The study in question looked at 25,714 adult men who were followed for approximately 10 years (2). During this time, there were 1,025 deaths among these men. The least fit 20% of men in each age group were considered to be the "low fitness" group. Men who were normal weight but were in the low fitness group had a 60% increased risk of dying from any cause. Men who were overweight and in the low fitness category had a 70% increased risk of death. Men who were obese and in the low fitness category had 230% increased risk of dying from any cause. Obesity and low physical activity—talk about your 1-2 combination!

The Nurses' Health Study

In 2004, researchers from Harvard published a study in the *New England Journal of Medicine* that examined the association between physical activity and all cause mortality in the Nurses' Health Study (3). This investigation included 116,564 women who were followed for 24 years. During this time, there were 10,282 deaths among these women.

When compared to women who engaged in physical activity for greater than three and a half hours per week, women with less than one hour of physical activity per week had a 55% increased risk of death. If the women were overweight (BMI 25-29.9) and were physically active for less than one hour per week, the increased risk of death rose to 64%. Finally, if the women were obese (BMI >30) and were physically active for less than one hour per week, they had a 240% increased risk of dying from any cause. As with the Cooper cohort, being sedentary and overweight was a dangerous combination, and normally these two lifestyle factors go hand in hand.

Heart Disease

The association between physical activity and coronary heart disease was examined in the Nurses' Health Study in 2006 (4). This study included 88,393 women who were followed for 20 years. During this time there were 2,358 major coronary events. This number included both fatal heart disease and non-fatal myocardial infarction.

Increasing physical activity resulted in a graded decrease in risk of heart disease. When compared to women who exercised for three and a half hours per week or more, women who exercised between one and three and a half hours per week had a 43% increased risk of coronary heart disease. Women who exercised for less than one hour per week had a 58% increased risk of heart disease.

Stroke

The association between physical activity and risk of stroke was examined in 72,488 women from the Nurses' Health Study. These women were followed for 8 years during which time there were 407 strokes (5). Women who exercised the most had a 34% lower risk of stroke when compared to women who exercised the least. The researchers thought the benefit was due to a lower blood pressure, higher HDL cholesterol level, improved blood clotting, improved insulin sensitivity, and better weight maintenance among the exercisers.

Cancer

A number of studies have shown a protective effect of physical activity on risk of cancer. We'll take a look at two of these: colon and breast cancer.

Colon Cancer

The association between physical activity and colon cancer was examined in the Health Professional Follow-up Study. Over 47,700 men were followed for six years with 203 cases of colon cancer and 586 adenomas emerging during this time period (6). Men who exercised the most had a 47% lower risk of colon cancer when compared to men who exercised the least. The researchers hypothesized that high insulin levels may have accounted for the difference in risk. High insulin is related to both a sedentary lifestyle as well as the growth of colonic mucosal cells. Physical activity also stimulates colonic motility, which may explain the reduced risk among the exercisers.

Breast Cancer

The association between physical activity and breast cancer was examined in 85,364 women from the Nurses' Health Study (7). After 16 years of follow-up, there were 3,137 new cases of breast cancer diagnosed among these women. Subjects who exercised an average of seven hours a week or more had an 18% lower risk of breast cancer than those who exercised for less than one hour per week. The researchers hypothesized that physical activity may act to reduce the risk of breast cancer by reducing exposure to circulating ovarian hormones.

Diabetes

Harvard researchers looked at the connection between physical activity and type 2 diabetes in 37,918 men from the Health Professional Follow-up Study (8). After 10 years of follow-up, 1,058 men were diagnosed with type 2 diabetes. The men who exercised the most had half the risk of diabetes compared to men who exercised the least. The researchers believed the protective effects of exercise were due to a lower weight and a more favorable body fat distribution among the exercisers. Physical activity is inversely associated with visceral fat, and less visceral fat means less insulin resistance.

Cognitive Function

The association between physical activity and cognitive function was examined in 18,766 women from the Nurses' Health Study (9). Women reported physical activity on a biennial mailed questionnaire and completed validated telephone cognitive assessments two years apart. The tests measured general cognition, verbal memory, category fluency, and attention.

Higher levels of physical activity were associated with better cognitive performance. Furthermore, women with the most physical activity had a 20% lower risk of cognitive impairment. The benefit was found for high intensity physical activity as well as moderate intensity physical activity such as brisk walking. The protective effects of exercise were thought to be due to lower blood pressure, improved lipoprotein profiles, decreased insulin resistance, and more adequate cerebral perfusion among the exercisers.

Weight Maintenance

As many of you likely know from personal experience, losing weight is tough, but keeping it off is even harder. Physical activity has been shown to help keep the weight you lose from coming back.

The association between physical activity and weight regain was examined in 4,558 women from the

Nurses' Health Study II cohort (10). All of the women included in this investigation had lost greater than 5% of their body weight in the two years prior to the start of this study. Weight regain was defined as gaining back at least 30% of their lost weight. Women who exercised for 30 or more minutes each day decreased their risk of weight regain by 31%.

Designing Your Physical Activity Program

Before getting started on any physical activity program, I strongly recommend that you mention to your doctor that you are about to start an exercise program and want to make sure you are medically cleared to do so. This is very important, and often I will not recommend any exercise for a new client until I receive medical clearance that it is safe to do so.

Once you've gotten the OK from your doc, you'll want to focus on two separate areas when designing your physical activity program: resistance training and cardiovascular exercise. Resistance training is important to maintain and even add to your metabolically active muscle tissue. This will make it easier to manage your weight and stay active until a ripe old age. In fact, most of what we associate with aging is actually the loss of lean muscle tissue.

Cardiovascular exercise is where you will burn your calories. Burning calories is pivotal to weight maintenance. Cardio will also allow you to reap all of the health benefits mentioned in this chapter. No fitness routine is complete without each of these two components.

Resistance Training

Once we hit our 25th birthday, we start to lose muscle at the rate of about 1% per year. This is a natural part of the aging process. This is troubling because each and every pound of muscle burns 50 calories per day, so as we lose this muscle, our metabolism drops and we gain weight.

Hitting the weights at least twice a week will prevent this loss of lean tissue. Now, I am not a body builder, and I don't advocate lifting heavy weights at all. Focus on lighter weights and higher repetitions. Make sure you do one exercise for your back, chest, shoulders, biceps, triceps, legs, and abs. If you are unsure of how to do this, consider hiring a personal trainer for a session or two to teach you the basics and then you'll be off and running.

A basic program should take you no more than 20 or 30 minutes to complete, and generally you can workout right at home. All you'll need is an exercise mat and some dumbbells. Again, twice a week for 20-30 minutes will greatly help reduce the loss of lean tissue and keep your metabolism burning calories.

Cardiovascular Exercise

There are three areas of a cardiovascular exercise program that need attention: type, duration, and most importantly, intensity.

Type

The type of cardio that you choose should be based on what you like to do, what you'll stick to, as well as your specific fitness goals.

Types Of Cardiovascular Exercise

Walking	Walking/Jogging
Biking	Rowing
Stairmaster	Elliptical Training
Swimming	Ice Skating
Roller Blading	Aerobic Dance

If your goal is to improve fitness and reduce the risk of disease, any of the above exercises will fit the bill. If you are a bit older or out of shape, brisk walking is a great start. As you become more fit, you may want to try some of the other more intense forms of cardiovascular exercise. These will give you more bang for your fitness buck than walking. When trying a new, more intense exercise, start slow and listen to your body.

If your goal is weight loss, I'd go with elliptical training, stair climbing or a modified jog/walk program (jog for two minutes and then walk for three minutes). These forms of cardio are weight supported, and you'll burn more calories with these than with the other forms of exercise. I don't recommend running under any circumstances. It is just too high impact. When you run, you put up to 6 times your body weight on your joints. Over time, this will likely cause orthopedic injuries. The majority of my clients use the elliptical trainer and get amazing results with much less stress on their joints.

Duration/Frequency

So how much exercise do we need? If your goal is to improve your health and reduce your risk of disease, I'd look no further than the 2008 Physical Activity Guidelines for Americans (1). According to these recommendations, 150 minutes per week of brisk walking or 75 minutes per week of more vigorous exercise will greatly improve fitness and decrease the risk of today's most deadly diseases. I'd definitely go more toward the 150 minutes per week.

If your goal is weight loss, you'll have to do more. Studies done in the Nurses' Health Study and the National Weight Control Registry show that in order to lose weight, you'll have to ramp up the cardio. I tell my weight loss clients (particularly my female clients) to shoot for 250 minutes of cardio per week. Again, I have them focus on an upright, weight bearing form of cardio like jogging/walking intervals, stair climbing, or better yet, elliptical training. With these exercises you are truly maximizing calories burned while protecting your joints from injury.

Intensity

If your goal is to reduce risk of disease, don't worry too much about your intensity. Just get out and get moving. Terrific health benefits have been documented for even moderate forms of physical activity like walking.

If your goal is weight loss, you'll have to focus a bit more on your intensity. A great way to tell that you are working hard enough is the sweat test. After five minutes into your cardio session, you should be sweating. If not, ramp it up! You want to be working at a level of 7 out of 10, with 10 being an all out sprint. Another great way to measure intensity is the talk test. When working at the proper intensity for weight loss, you should need to take a breath after a normal length sentence. If you can get two or three sentences out without taking a breath, pick up the pace. If you are taking a breath after every other word, slow it down a bit.

TAKE HOME MESSAGE

1) Humans were meant to be physically active.
2) Physical activity helps reduce the risk of most major diseases, including heart disease, stroke, diabetes, cancer, Alzheimer's, and cognitive dysfunction.
3) Pick a form of physical activity and get moving!
4) If your goal is general health, shoot for 150 minutes per week.
5) If your goal is weight loss, shoot for 250 minutes per week and pick an upright and more intense method of physical activity like elliptical training.
6) Include resistance training at least twice per week to build muscle and increase metabolic rate.

References

1) U.S. Dept. of Health and Human Services. 2008 Physical Activity Guidelines For Americans.

2) Wei M, Kampert JB, Barlow CE, et al. Relationship between low cardiorespiratory fitness and mortality in normal weight, overweight, and obese men. *Journal of the American Medical Association* 1999; 282:1547-1553.

3) Hu FB, Willett WC, Li T, et al. Adiposity as compared with physical activity in predicting mortality among women. *New England Journal of Medicine* 2004; 351:2694-2703.

4) Li TY, Rana JS, Manson JE, et al. Obesity as compared with physical activity in predicting risk of coronary heart disease in women. *Circulation* 2006; 113:499-506.

5) Hu FB, Stampfer MJ, Colditz GA, et al. Physical activity and risk of stroke in women. *Journal of the American Medical Association* 2000; 283:2961-67.

6) Giovannucci E, Ascherio A, Rimm EB, et al. Physical activity, obesity, and risk for colon cancer and adenoma in men. *Annals of Internal Medicine* 1995; 122:327-334.

7) Rockhill B, Willett WC, Hunter DJ, et al. A prospective study of recreational physical activity and breast cancer risk. *Archives of Internal Medicine* 1999; 159:2290-2296.

8) Hu FB, Leitzmann MF, Stampfer MJ, et al. Physical activity and television watching in relation to risk for type 2 diabetes mellitus in men. *Archives of Internal Medicine* 2001; 161:1542-48.

9) Weuve J, Kang JH, Manson JE, et al. Physical activity, including walking, and cognitive function in older women. *Journal of the American Medical Association* 2004; 292:1454-61.

10) Mekary RA, Feskanich D, Hu FB, et al. Physical activity in relation to long-term weight maintenance after intentional weight loss in premenopausal women. *Obesity* 2009; 18:167-74.

Priority #4
Choose Low Glycemic Load Carbohydrates

The type of carbohydrate that you put into your body can have a major impact on your risk of disease. Americans are currently choosing way too many of the wrong carbohydrates and way too few of the right ones. Chances are, you are too. Let's start from the top. What is a carbohydrate? Carbohydrates are composed of carbon, hydrogen, and oxygen in the ratio of 1:2:1. The main function of carbohydrates is to provide energy for the body and to prevent the breakdown of protein.

The type of carbohydrates that humans have consumed has changed dramatically over the years. While we were evolving, the majority of the carbohydrates we ate were fruits and vegetables in their whole form, beans and other legumes, and grains that were highly unrefined. As we became more civilized, this all changed—for the worse!

Before refrigeration, the transport and storage of food was a big problem. Whole grains contain a small amount of fat. This fat shortens the amount of time it takes for the grain to spoil. Therefore, early attempts to refine grains were initiated by the noblest of intentions—to keep food edible longer so fewer people would starve. Unfortunately, refining grains dramatically alters the way our body handles the carbohydrate during digestion.

Biochemistry 101

Let's go over a brief lesson on what happens to your blood sugar when you eat a carbohydrate. Once you consume a carbohydrate, your blood sugar levels begin to rise. Our body works within a relatively narrow frame of blood sugar. You've got a problem if it goes too high, and you've got a problem if it goes too low. For this reason, the body releases insulin to lower your blood sugar. The amount of insulin released depends on the type and the amount of carbohydrate consumed. Some carbohydrates cause the release of a large amount of insulin, while others cause a smaller amount of insulin to be released.

This peak in blood sugar and insulin levels can have a dramatic impact on our health when we choose the wrong type of carbohydrate. In summary, not all carbs are created equal. Some spike your blood sugar and insulin levels and some have a more modest effect.

Enter the glycemic index. The glycemic index was proposed by Dr. David Jenkins from the University of Toronto in 1981 as a way of classifying carbohydrates. Very simply, it gives a score as to how quickly and how severely a carbohydrate will raise your blood sugar. It all starts by feeding a group of subjects 50 grams of glucose (which is pure sugar) and measuring their blood sugar response. Next, the researchers feed the same people 50 grams of another type of carbohydrate, say a baked potato, and then measure their blood sugar response once again.

The glycemic index number is the blood sugar response of that particular carb relative to the pure glucose reading. For example, the glycemic index of a white baked potato is 78. What this really means is that when you eat equal amounts of a white baked potato and pure glucose, the potato results in 78% of the blood sugar response of the pure glucose. This test is repeated for all types of carbohydrate containing foods.

Take a look at this example. Notice how the higher glycemic carbohydrate causes dramatic increases in insulin and glucose levels compared to the lower glycemic carbohydrate.

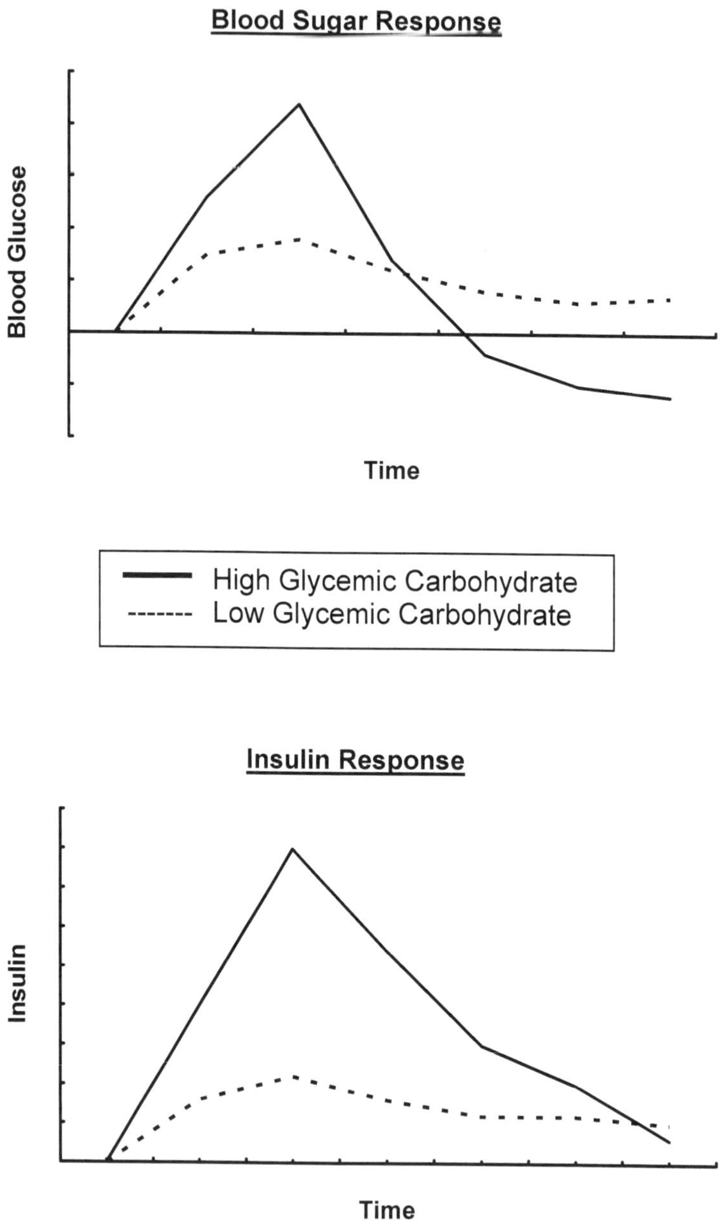
Blood Sugar Response
Blood Glucose
Time
High Glycemic Carbohydrate
Low Glycemic Carbohydrate
Insulin Response
Insulin
Time

A related concept is the glycemic load. The glycemic load of a food was proposed by some of my colleagues at Harvard University. The glycemic load is the glycemic index multiplied by the amount of carbohydrate supplied in a typical serving of the food. So, the glycemic load takes into account both the quality and the quantity of a carbohydrate.

Why is this important? Well, for starters, the glycemic load gives you a more practical look at how much a carbohydrate will affect your blood sugar. Most of the foods that have a high glycemic index also have a high glycemic load. For example, white rice has a glycemic index of 91 (very high) and a glycemic load of 24.8 (also considered very high). White bread has a glycemic index of 70 and a glycemic load of 21, both considered high. On the other end of the spectrum, lentils have a low glycemic index of 29 and a low glycemic load of 5.7. Apples similarly have a low glycemic index (36) and a low glycemic load (8.1).

However, there are some interesting exceptions. Carrots have a high glycemic index at 71, but the glycemic load of carrots is small, at 3.8. This is because carrots have a lot of fiber and water and supply only a small amount of carbohydrate per serving. Hence the lower glycemic load. Remember, glycemic load is the product of both the glycemic index and the amount of carbohydrate.

So, you can see that some foods with a high glycemic index really won't hurt your blood sugar (because only small amounts of carbs are delivered).

Other foods with more moderate glycemic indices (like pasta) will really hurt your blood sugar because of the large amount of carbohydrates delivered in a serving. To improve your health and reduce your risk of disease, you want to focus on foods with a low glycemic load.

It should not come as a surprise that the overwhelming majority of foods with a high glycemic load are man-made, refined carbohydrates. The big offenders are bread, pasta, white rice, and sugar. This makes sense because fruits, vegetables, and legumes are the carbohydrates that were put on this Earth for us to consume. These are the foods we evolved with, and it is not surprising that our bodies function best when consuming them.

Examples Of Higher And Lower Glycemic Load Foods

Higher Glycemic Load	Lower Glycemic Load
White bread	Fruits
White rice	Vegetables
Pasta	Legumes
Sugar	Oatmeal
White potatoes	Brown Rice

Foods with a high glycemic index and/or load have been associated with a variety of disease outcomes. Let's see what the research says about the impact of high glycemic foods on our health.

Heart Disease

The Nurses' Health Study

I personally published a paper in 2006 that examined the association between glycemic load and risk of coronary heart disease in women from the Nurses' Health Study. We followed 82,802 women for 20 years, during which time there were 1,994 new cases of coronary heart disease (1). Women with the highest dietary glycemic load had a 90% increased risk of coronary heart disease compared to women with the lowest dietary glycemic load. We theorized that the increased risk was due to the negative impact on HDL cholesterol, triglycerides, and insulin sensitivity that is often seen with high glycemic load diets.

European Prospective Investigation Into Cancer and Nutrition Cohort

The association between glyemic index, glycemic load, and cardiovascular disease was examined in 15,714 Dutch women from the EPIC cohort (2). The women were followed for nine years, during which time there were 556 new cases of coronary heart disease and 243 cases of cerebrovascular accident (stroke).

Women with the highest dietary glyemic load had a 47% increased risk of cardiovascular disease when compared to women with the lowest dietary glycemic load. Similarly, women with the highest glycemic index had a 33% increased risk of cardiovascular disease when compared to women with the lowest glycemic index. The results were particularly pronounced in overweight women. The researchers attributed the increased risk to the detrimental effects of high glycemic diets on insulin sensitivity and blood lipid profiles.

Stroke

The association between dietary glycemic load and risk of stroke was examined in the Nurses' Health Study in 2005 (3). Over 78,700 women were followed for 18 years, during which time there were 1,020 new cases of stroke. Among women with a BMI of 25 or higher, dietary glycemic load was associated with a 61% increased risk of stroke. This association was not seen in women of normal weight. The combination of a high glycemic load diet and overweight seemed to be the most harmful. The researchers theorized that the increased risk seen with the higher glycemic diet was due to decreases in HDL cholesterol, increases in blood pressure, C-reactive protein, and insulin resistance. All of these factors tend to increase risk of stroke.

Cancer

The association between glycemic load and colon cancer was assessed in the Women's Health Study cohort (4). Over 38,450 women were followed for eight years, and during this time there were 174 new cases of colon cancer. Women with the highest dietary glycemic load had almost 3 times the risk of developing colon cancer when compared to women with the lowest glycemic load. The researchers believed the higher rate of cancer was due to higher insulin and insulin derived growth factor levels in women with the higher glycemic load diets. These hormones are thought to stimulate mitosis and cell proliferation.

Type 2 Diabetes

During my years at Harvard, I published a study that looked at the association between glycemic load and risk of type 2 diabetes in the Nurses' Health Study (5). We looked at 85,059 women over 20 years. During this time, there were 4,670 new cases of type 2 diabetes. Women with the highest dietary glycemic load had 2½ times the risk of type 2 diabetes when compared to women with the lowest dietary glycemic load. We hypothesized that the lower glycemic load diet offered protection due to its decreased glucose and insulin response, lowered glycated hemoglobin, and improved insulin sensitivity.

Weight Loss

Several randomized trials have been conducted recently to examine the effects of low glycemic diets on weight loss. Here are two of the most notable:

In 2007, a trial was published in the *American Journal of Clinical Nutrition* that randomly assigned 86 subjects into one of two diet groups. Forty-three subjects were assigned to a reduced glyemic load diet, and the other 43 were assigned to a low fat diet (6). By the end of 12 weeks, those assigned to the reduced glycemic load diet lost significantly more weight (10.8 lbs. vs 5.5 lbs). By the end of 36 weeks, the difference in weight between the two groups was not significant statistically, but the lower glycemic load group was still down about 4 lbs compared to the low fat group.

Another trial was published in 2007 in the *Journal of the American Medical Association* (7). This investigation compared the effects of a low glycemic load diet versus a low fat diet on body weight. Changes in body weight did not differ in the groups overall after 18 months. However, in those with higher insulin levels at baseline, the lower glycemic load group lost significantly more weight (12.8 lbs v 2.6 lbs) and body fat (2.6% vs 0.9%). This study provides more evidence that the effects of a high glycemic load diet appear to be more important for those who are overweight and therefore are more likely to be insulin resistant. Currently, two out of three Americans would fall into this category.

Recommendations On Carbohydrates

OK, so how does one avoid the perils of a high glycemic load diet and enjoy the benefits of a lower glycemic load diet? There are actually three strategies to lower the glyemic load of your diet. Before we get to that, you need to remember that the glycemic load of your diet is influenced by both the quality of the carbohydrate that you consume and the total amount of carbohydrate that you consume.

Strategy 1: Limit High Glycemic Load Carbs

The first strategy is to strictly limit those carbohydrates that will result in the highest peak blood glucose and insulin levels. Generally these foods are: bread in all of its forms, white rice, pasta, sugar, and white potatoes. I know that it sounds tough to eliminate these foods from your diet. Keep in mind that after a couple of weeks, you'll actually stop craving them. Cravings for refined carbs are far more physiological than psychological. I've seen this with my clients for 15 years. Stabilize the blood sugar and the cravings go away. Following is a list of the carbs you'll want to strictly limit:

Carbohydrates To Avoid

White Bread	Other Fruit Juice
Wheat Bread	Soda
Tortillas	Cakes
Wraps	Cookies
Pita Bread	Pies
Pasta	Candy
White Rice	Donuts
Bananas	Ketchup
Grapes	BBQ Sauce
White Potatoes	Steak Sauce
Crackers	Jams
Rice Cakes	Jellies
Popcorn	Sweetened Yogurt
Bagels	Raisins
Pretzels	Other Dried Fruit
Potato Chips	Low Fat Salad Dressing
Sugar	Anything Else With Sugar!!!
Orange Juice	
Tomato Juice	

Strategy #2: Eat Low Glycemic Load Carbs

If most of the carbs you consume come from natural, whole foods, you are well on your way to lowering the glycemic load of your diet. Focus on fruits, vegetables, legumes (like black beans, lentils, and hummus), brown rice, and old fashioned oatmeal (not instant or quick) for your carbs. Following is a more comprehensive list of the right carbohydrates to pick:

Best Choices For Carbohydrates

Apples	Green Pepper
Oranges	Red Pepper
Pineapple	Olives
Blueberries	Carrots
Strawberries	Spinach
Raspberries	Lettuce
Melon	Peas
Grapefruit	Lentils
Watermelon	Black Beans
Mango	Pink Beans
Papaya	Chick Peas
Kiwi	Hummus
Sweet Potato	Other Beans
Broccoli	Other Fruits
Cauliflower	Other Vegetables
Tomatoes	Brown Rice
Brussels Sprouts	Quinoa
Onion	Oatmeal (Not Instant)
Radishes	

Strategy #3: Go Easy On The Carbs

Aim for a moderate carbohydrate consumption. Remember, the glycemic load of your diet is affected by both the quality of the carbohydrate you eat as well as the amount. Even if you are eating healthy carbs, if you take in too many, you'll raise your glycemic load. A great way to moderate your carbohydrate levels is to eat more lean protein (like chicken, turkey, seafood, legumes, eggs) and more healthy vegetable fats (like olive oil, canola oil, nuts, seeds, avocados). I have my clients shoot for roughly 40-45% carbohydrate, 20-25% lean protein and 35-40% healthy fat. Don't get too caught up in the numbers, just make sure you are eating a good amount of protein at each meal, a moderate serving of healthy fat and then add in your healthy, low glycemic carbs.

Another benefit to eating a source of fat, protein, and carbohydrate at each meal is that the fat and protein slow the entry of carbohydrate into the blood stream. This acts to slow the absorption of the carbohydrate which results in less of a blood sugar spike.

If you eat this way, you will lower your glycemic and insulin response while still benefiting from all of the healthful properties of carbohydrates in the diet. These benefits include their high fiber, vitamin, mineral, and cancer fighting phytochemical content.

This is considered a more Mediterranean style diet, and you will notice a number of other benefits when eating this way. Your energy will improve, you will have an easier time maintaining your weight because you'll be far less hungry, and you'll even improve your mood. Swings in blood sugar can leave you tired, irritable, and stressed out.

TAKE HOME MESSAGE:

1) The type of carbohydrate you consume can have a dramatic impact on your health.
2) Some carbs spike your blood sugar and insulin to unnaturally high levels. These are known as high glycemic load carbs.
3) Low glycemic load carbs have a more moderate affect on blood sugar and insulin levels.
4) High glycemic load carbs have been associated with heart disease, stroke, some cancers, type 2 diabetes, and weight gain.
5) To lower the glycemic load of your diet, pick carbs like fruits, vegetables, legumes, brown rice, and oatmeal while limiting intakes of white bread, pasta, white rice, and sugar.
6) Eat a moderate amount of carbohydrates and include a healthy dose of lean protein and vegetable fat with each meal.

References

1) Halton TL, Willett WC, Liu S, et al. Low carbohydrate diet score and the risk of coronary heart disease in women. *New England Journal of Medicine* 2006; 355:1991-2002.

2) Buelens JW, De Bruijne LM, Stolk RP, et al. High dietary glycemic load and glycemic index increase risk of cardiovascular disease among middle aged women: A population based follow up study. *Journal of the American College of Cardiology* 2007; 50:14-21.

3) Oh K, Hu FB, Cho E, et al. Carbohydrate intake, glycemic index, glycemic load, and dietary fiber in relation to risk of stroke in women. *American Journal of Epidemiology* 2005; 161:161-69.

4) Higginbotham S, Zhang ZF, Lee IM, et al. Dietary glycemic load and risk of colorectal cancer in the Women's Health Study. *Journal of the National Cancer Institute* 2004; 96:229-33.

5) Halton TL, Liu S, Manson JE, et al. Low carbohydrate diet score and risk of type 2 diabetes in women. *American Journal Of Clinical Nutrition* 2008; 87:339-46.

6) Maki KC, Rains TM, Kaden VN, et al. Effects of a reduced glycemic load diet on body weight, body composition, and cardiovascular disease risk markers in overweight and obese adults. *American Journal of Clinical Nutrition* 2007; 85:724-34.

7) Ebbeling CB, Leidig MM, Feldman HA, et al. Effects of a low glycemic load vs low fat diet in obese young adults. *Journal of the American Medical Association* 2007; 297:2092-2102.

Priority# 5
Pick Your Fats Carefully

Fat is without a doubt, the most misunderstood nutrient in the field of nutrition. Fats, also known as lipids, are a wide variety of compounds that share one common trait: they don't dissolve readily in water. Lipids that are solid at room temperature (like butter) are called fats. Lipids that are liquid at room temperature are called oils (like canola oil).

Some of the major functions of fat include:

1) Providing energy for the body.
2) Storing energy for the body.
3) Insulating and protecting vital organs.
4) Transportation of the fat soluble vitamins A, D, E, and K.

Dietary fat has gotten a *bad reputation!* Early nutrition research showed that certain fats were associated with an increased risk of cancer and heart disease. Another knock against fat is that it is very calorie dense, providing 9 calories per gram. For these reasons, the main thrust of nutrition advice in the 1980's and 1990's was to drastically reduce the amount of fat in our diets. The motivating force behind this advice was to prevent a variety of diseases and decrease the incidence of obesity.

However, making such a blanket recommendation concerning dietary fat was akin to throwing the baby out with the bath water. It turns out that the amount of fat in your diet is not associated with weight gain, and although some fats increase the risk of major diseases, others reduce the risk of those same diseases.

OK, so what are the good fats and what are the bad fats? Let's describe each of the types of fats quickly and then take a look at what the research tells us about their impact on our health.

Saturated Fat

Saturated fats are fats that contain no double bonds. All of the carbons are saturated with hydrogen. They are found, for the most part, in animal products. They are found in high amounts in fatty cuts of red meat like steak, bacon, hot dogs, butter, and full fat dairy products like cheese, ice cream, and whole milk. These are considered bad fats due to their negative impact on our health.

Trans Fat

Trans fat is actually a man-made fat. It is produced through the commercial hydrogenation of polyunsaturated oils. This is done to increase the shelf life of food items and to improve the texture and mouth feel of the food. Trans fats are found in commercially prepared oils used to fry foods and in baked goods and some margarines. In the last couple of years, the dangers of trans fats have become much more widely known, and their use has decreased considerably. However, they are still out there, and as you'll learn, trans fat is a very deadly fat.

Monounsaturated Fat

Monounsaturated fats have a slightly different structure than other fats; they contain one double bond, so not all of their carbons are saturated with hydrogen. You'll find these fats in olive oil, canola oil, as well as a variety of nuts and avocados. These are considered a healthy fat.

Polyunsaturated Fat

Polyunsaturated fats are highly similar to monounsaturated fats, but instead of having just one double bond, they have two or more. These fats are found in most nuts and plant oils like corn, soybean, and safflower oil. These fats are considered healthy.

Now let's take a look at what the research tells us about how these different fats impact our health.

Heart Disease

Each of the four types of fats was examined for their association with heart disease in over 80,000 women from the Nurses' Health Study. After 14 years of follow-up, there were 939 cases of fatal heart disease and non-fatal myocardial infarction (1). Following are some of the major findings of this important paper:

- Each increase of 5% of energy as saturated fat was associated with a 17% increased risk of heart disease as compared to a 5% increase in carbohydrates.
- A 2% increase in energy as trans fat was associated with a 93% increased risk of heart disease compared to equivalent energy from carbohydrate.
- A 5% increase in energy from monounsaturated fat was associated with a 19% decreased risk of heart disease.
- A 5% increase in energy from polyunsaturated fat was associated with a 38% decreased risk of coronary heart disease.
- Total fat was not associated with risk of heart disease.

In summary, saturated fat was found to be moderately harmful when it comes to risk of heart disease, trans fat was very harmful, while monounsaturated and polyunsaturated fat offered protection. Most of the effects of the four fats on risk of heart disease were thought to be due to their influence on serum cholesterol.

Saturated fats tend to raise LDL cholesterol, which is known to increase risk of heart disease. Trans fat raises LDL and lowers HDL cholesterol (the beneficial cholesterol). This is a like a one-two combination and is very harmful. Monounsaturated and polyunsaturated fats tend to have a favorable effect on blood cholesterol by decreasing LDL and raising HDL cholesterol.

Type 2 Diabetes

The association between different types of fats and risk of type 2 diabetes was also examined in the Nurses' Health Study. Over 84,200 women were followed for 14 years, and during this time there were 2,507 new cases of type 2 diabetes (2). Total fat, monounsaturated fat, and saturated fat were not associated with risk of type 2 diabetes. However, a 2% increase in trans fat consumption resulted in a 39% increased risk of type 2 diabetes. A 5% increase in polyunsaturated fat was associated with a 37% decreased risk of type 2 diabetes.

The researchers believed that the benefit of polyunsaturated fat was due to improved insulin sensitivity. Similarly, the damaging effects of trans fat were thought to be due to its negative impact on insulin sensitivity.

Cancer

Although there is not clear evidence of a relationship between different types of fat and cancer, there have been a few relevant studies that suggest one may exist.

Breast Cancer

The association between dietary fat and breast cancer was examined in the Nurses' Health Study II cohort. Over 90,650 pre-menopausal women (between the ages of 26-46) were followed for eight years (3). During this time, there were 714 new cases of invasive breast cancer. Women with the highest animal fat intake had a 33% increased risk of breast cancer. Both red meat and high fat dairy were associated with an increased risk of breast cancer. Vegetable fat was not associated with risk of breast cancer.

The researchers believed that heterocyclic amines may have been the reason for the increased risk associated with red meat consumption. Thesc carcinogenic substances are formed when red meat is cooked at a high temperature. Growth factors found in high fat dairy were thought to be the causative factor in the relationship between high fat dairy products and risk of breast cancer.

Prostate Cancer

The association between dietary fat and risk of prostate cancer was examined in the Health Professional Follow-up Study. Over 47,800 men were followed for four years, during which time there were 300 new cases of prostate cancer (4). Total fat consumption was directly related to risk of prostate cancer. Men who consumed the most fat had a 79% increased risk when compared to men who consumed the least fat.

These results seem to have been driven by animal fat, which was also independently related to risk of prostate cancer (a 63% increased risk for those consuming the most animal fat). However, this association was not statistically significant. Red meat was strongly related to the risk of prostate cancer with the men consuming the most red meat (30.5 grams per day) having a 250% increased risk of prostate cancer when compared to men who consumed the least (3.2 grams per day). Vegetable fat was not related to risk of prostate cancer. Carcinogens formed during the cooking of red meat seemed to be the mechanism behind the increased risk.

Non-Hodgkin's Lymphoma

The association between dietary fat and non-Hodgkin's lymphoma was examined in 88,410 women in the Nurses' Health Study (5). During 14 years of follow-up, there were 199 new cases of non-Hodgkin's lymphoma. Women who consumed the most trans fat (3.2% of energy) had 2.4 times the risk of developing the disease when compared to women with the lowest intakes of trans fat (1.3% of energy).

Omega 3 Fatty Acids

Omega 3 fatty acids are a very special polyunsaturated fatty acid that has been shown to have a powerfully beneficial impact on our health. They are found in fish, canola oil, soybean oil, and walnuts.

Several studies have examined the affects of omega 3's on our risk of disease.

Omega 3 Fatty Acids and Heart Disease

The association between omega 3 fatty acids and risk of coronary heart disease was examined in 84,688 women from the Nurses' Health Study (6). The nurses were followed for 16 years, during which time there were 1,513 new cases of coronary heart disease. Women with the highest intake of omega 3 fatty acids had a 33% decreased risk of coronary heart disease when compared to women with the lowest intake. The protective effects of the omega 3 fatty acids were thought to be the result of their beneficial impact on triglycerides, platelet aggregability, and their anti-arrhythmic effects.

Omega 3 Fatty Acids And Stroke

The association between omega 3 fatty acids and risk of stroke was also examined in 79,839 women in the Nurses' Health Study (7). Women were followed for 14 years, during which time there were 574 strokes in this cohort. Women with the highest omega 3 consumption had a 28% lower risk of stroke when compared to women with the lowest intake of omega 3's. The benefit was thought to be due to omega 3's positive impact on platelet aggregability, vasodilation, blood pressure, insulin levels, and plasma fibrinogen.

Nuts

Nuts are a really good source of healthy fat, and several studies have looked at the association between nuts and risk of disease. Here is a sampling of this research:

Nuts And Coronary Heart Disease

The association between nut consumption and coronary heart disease was examined in 86,016 women from the Nurses' Health Study (8). After 14 years of follow-up, there were 1,255 coronary events in this cohort. Women who consumed more than five ounces of nuts per week had a 35% lower risk of heart disease than those who ate less than one ounce of nuts per month. The benefit was thought to come from the nuts' positive impact on serum cholesterol levels.

Nuts And Type 2 Diabetes

The association between nut consumption and type 2 diabetes was examined in 83,818 women from the Nurses' Health Study (9). During 16 years of follow-up, there were 3,206 new cases of type 2 diabetes in this cohort. Women who ate nuts greater or equal to five times per week had a 27% decreased risk of type 2 diabetes compared to women who rarely ate nuts. The beneficial effects of nuts were thought to be due to their positive impact on insulin sensitivity. Nuts are also good sources of fiber, magnesium, vitamins, minerals, antioxidants, and plant proteins. Each of these has also been shown to reduce the risk of type 2 diabetes.

Recommendations On Fats

1) *Don't Go Low Fat*—Research has shown that certain fats are quite health promoting. Therefore, there is no reason to eat a low fat diet. Fat also provides satiety, so you'll be much less hungry when you include some in each meal. When healthy fat replaces carbohydrate in your diet, it will also act to lower your overall glycemic load. We learned why this is important in the last chapter. I have my clients shoot for about 35% of their calories as healthy fat.

2) *Limit Saturated Fat And Avoid Trans Fat*—These fats have a negative impact on our health. Trans fats must now legally be listed on food labels so they are really easy to find. Try to limit trans fat to 0 grams per day and saturated fat to at most 7% of calories. Check out the list of fats to avoid on the next page.

3) *Focus On Poly- And Monounsaturated Fats*—These fats are extremely health promoting and should not be avoided, but enjoyed. Check out the list of healthy fats on the next page.

Fats To Avoid

Whole Milk	Hamburger
Whole Cheese	Bologna
Whole Yogurt	Pepperoni
Whole Cottage Cheese	Pastrami
Ice Cream	Steak
Butter	Salami
Margarine	Snack Chips
Palm Oil	Pies
Coconut Oil	Cakes
Hot Dogs	Cookies
Sausage	Crackers
Bacon	Chocolate
Cream	Any Trans Fat

Fats To Focus On

Olive Oil	Pistachios
Canola Oil	Macadamia Nuts
Corn Oil	Any Other Nut
Sunflower Oil	Sunflower Seeds
Safflower Oil	Pumpkin Seeds
Soybean Oil	Avocados
Flaxseed Oil	Peanut Butter
Other Vegetable Oils	Almond Butter
Peanuts	Cashew Butter
Almonds	Pistachio Butter
Walnuts	Smart Balance
Cashews	Olivio
Hazel Nuts	Mayonnaise

Although the right fats are health promoting, keep in mind that they are very calorie dense. Therefore, keep portions sensible so all of those extra calories don't push the scale in the wrong direction. Again, keeping fat to about 35% of calories is what we are looking for here.

TAKE HOME MESSAGE

1) Not all fats are the same, some are good for you, and some are bad for you.
2) Saturated fat and trans fat have been associated with an increased risk of chronic disease.
3) Polyunsaturated fat and monounsaturated fat have been associated with a decreased risk of chronic disease.
4) Don't be afraid of dietary fat! When you choose your fats wisely, they can decrease risk of disease, help stabilize your blood sugar, provide satiety after a meal, and lower the glycemic load of your diet.
5) Shoot for about 35% of your calories as dietary fat. Focus on the healthy fats from the list provided and limit the unhealthy fats from the list provided.

References

1) Hu FB, Stampfer MJ, Manson JE, et al. Dietary fat intake and risk of coronary heart disease in women. *New England Journal of Medicine* 1997; 337:1491–1499.

2) Salmeron J, Hu FB, Manson JE, et al. Dietary fat intake and risk of type 2 diabetes in women. *American Journal of Clinical Nutrition* 2001; 73:1019-26.

3) Cho E, Spiegelman D, Hunter DJ, et al. Premenopausal fat intake and risk of breast cancer. *Journal of the National Cancer Institute* 2003; 95:1079-85.

4) Giovannucci E, Rimm EB, Colditz GA, et al. A prospective study of dietary fat and risk of prostate cancer. *Journal of the National Cancer Institute* 1993; 85:1571-79.

5) Zhang S, Hunter DJ, Rosner BA, et al. Dietary fat and protein in relation to risk of Non-Hodgkin's lymphoma among women. *Journal of the National Cancer Institute* 1999; 91:1751-58.

6) Hu FB, Bronner L, Willett WC, et al. Fish and omega-3 fatty acid intake and risk of coronary heart disease in women. *Journal of the American Medical Association* 2002; 287:1815-1821.

7) Iso H, Rexrode KM, Stampfer MJ, et al. Intake of fish and omega-3 fatty acids and risk of stroke in women. *Journal of the American Medical Association* 2001;285:304-312.

8) Hu FB, Stampfer MJ, Manson JE, et al. Frequent nut consumption and risk of coronary heart disease in women: prospective cohort study. *British Medical Journal* 1998; 317:1341-45.

9) Jiang R, Manson JE, Stampfer MJ, et al. Nut and peanut butter consumption and risk of type 2 diabetes. *Journal of the American Medical Association* 2002; 288:2554-60.

Priority # 6
Limit Sodium In Your Diet

Next on our list is sodium. Sodium has been getting a lot of attention in the field of nutrition research lately. It used to be that you were told to lower your dietary sodium if you had high blood pressure. If you didn't, you didn't have to worry too much about it. My how times have changed! It is now clear that we all have to lower the amount of sodium in our diet. In recent research literature, sodium has been associated with a number of chronic diseases. Before we get to that, let's get a little background on salt and sodium.

The terms salt and sodium are not interchangeable. Sodium is a mineral that our body needs for a variety of processes. Salt is made up of both sodium and chloride, 40% of salt is sodium.

Getting some sodium in our diet is absolutely essential to our health. Some of the functions of sodium include: 1) Maintaining fluid balance. 2) Transmission of nerve impulses. 3) Contraction of muscle fiber. However, we don't need much sodium to accomplish these tasks because our body is extremely efficient at absorbing sodium in our food. In fact, we really only need about 100 milligrams of sodium per day (1). We get more than that, much more. The typical American consumes about 3,400 milligrams of sodium each day. This is 34 times what our body needs.

So where do we get all of this sodium? Almost all foods contain some sodium naturally. However, approximately 75% of the sodium we consume in the U.S. comes from processed foods (2). In fact, if we ate only unprocessed foods in their natural form, and added no salt from the shaker, we would consume about 500 mg of sodium per day (1).

All of this extra sodium takes a toll on our health. Sodium has been shown to increase blood pressure, and therefore has been associated with an increased risk of heart disease and stroke. Sodium has also been associated with osteoporosis, and may even increase risk of stomach cancer. Let's take a look at some of the research.

Sodium And Hypertension

A large number of research studies have shown that dietary sodium can have a dramatic influence on blood pressure. An example of one such study is the Dietary Approaches to Stop Hypertension (DASH) trial. In this randomized trial, 412 participants were given a healthy blood pressure lowering diet or a control diet which reflected typical American food consumption (3).

Once the diets were assigned, subjects were given a low sodium (1,150 mg), an intermediate sodium (2,300 mg), and a high sodium (3,450 mg) level for a period of time, and then blood pressure was measured. Reducing sodium from the high to the intermediate level reduced systolic blood pressure by 2.1 mm/hg for the control diet group and 1.3 mm/hg for the healthy diet group. Further reducing sodium from the intermediate level to the low sodium level caused an additional reduction of 4.6 mm/hg for the control group and 1.7 mm/hg for the healthy diet group. Diastolic blood pressure was also similarly reduced 1.6 mm/hg from high to low sodium intake for the healthy diet group and 3.5 mm/hg in the control group.

This study shows that salt can affect your blood pressure whether you are eating a healthy diet or an unhealthy diet. The decrease in blood pressure with sodium reduction was greater for those with existing hypertension, but was also significant for those with normal blood pressure. An excess of sodium pulls water out of cells, and this is the main mechanism by which it is thought to increase blood pressure.

Sodium, Heart Disease, And Stroke

High blood pressure is a major risk factor for heart disease and stroke. Therefore, it would make sense that sodium would be associated with an increased risk of these diseases. This is exactly what the research tells us. A meta-analysis is a type of study that combines data from several investigations and comes up with a summary estimate. Recently, a meta-analysis on the effects of salt intake on stroke and heart disease was published in the *British Medical Journal* (4).

This meta-analysis included data from 19 different cohorts that included 177,025 men and women and over 11,000 cardiovascular events. High salt intake was associated with a statistically significant 23% increased risk of stroke and a borderline significant 14% increased risk of cardiovascular disease.

The researchers believed that the blood pressure raising effect of sodium was responsible for the increased risk of stroke and cardiovascular disease in these cohorts. However, they also mentioned potential effects independent of blood pressure, including a negative impact on left ventricular mass, arterial stiffness, and renal function.

Sodium And Bone Health

There is also evidence that high salt intakes have a negative impact on bone health. A study published in *The American Journal of Clinical Nutrition* looked at this issue in 124 post-menopausal women over a 10 year period (5). Urinary sodium excretion was negatively correlated with changes in bone density in the intertrochanteric and total hip sites. This means that as sodium increased in the diet, bone health changed for the worse.

When sodium is excreted in the urine, calcium is excreted along with it. When the body then needs calcium for its metabolic processes, it will take it from bone. This is most likely why a high consumption of sodium has a negative impact on bone health. The researchers also figured out that by halving sodium consumption in this study population, bone health would be effected as positively as if consuming 891 milligrams of calcium each day.

Sodium And Gastric Cancer

Although there is not a large body of evidence that sodium increases the risk of gastric cancer, there are a few studies that suggest such an association may exist. A Japanese study was published in *The British Journal of Cancer* in 2004 (6). This investigation included 18,684 men and 20,381 women aged 40-59 who were studied for 11 years. During this time there were 486 new cases of gastric cancer.

Men with the highest sodium intake had over 2 times the risk of gastric cancer compared to men with the lowest sodium intake. No association was found in women. However, there were few diagnoses of gastric cancer among women, so statistical power for these estimates may have been too low to detect an association. Salt is hypothesized to damage mucosal barriers and lead to inflammation, erosion, and degeneration of the stomach. These changes may increase the risk of gastric cancer.

Recommendations For Sodium

Ok, so we've seen that sodium has the potential to raise blood pressure, increase risk of heart disease and stroke, damage our bones, and maybe even increase the risk of gastric cancer. We also know that as Americans, we consume way too much salt, around 3,400 milligrams on average.

The first recommendation is simply to become aware of how much sodium is in the foods that you are eating. This is easy to do because sodium is a nutrient that must appear, by law, on all food labels. Look at the food label below. The amount of sodium is circled and is displayed in milligrams.

Nutrition Facts

Serving Size 1/2 cup (57g)
Servings Per Container 15

Amount Per Serving	
Calories 230	Calories from Fat 100
	% Daily Value*
Total Fat 11g	**17%**
Saturated Fat 2g	**10%**
Trans Fat 0g	
Cholesterol 0mg	**0%**
Sodium 95mg	**4%**
Total Carbohydrate 32g	**11%**
Dietary Fiber 3g	**12%**
Sugars 18g	
Protein 5g	
Vitamin A 0%	• Vitamin C 0%
Calcium 4%	• Iron 10%

*Percent Daily Values are based on a 2,000 calorie diet. Your daily values may be higher or lower depending on your calorie needs:

	Calories	2,000	2,500
Total Fat	Less Than	65g	80g
Saturated Fat	Less Than	20g	25g
Cholesterol	Less Than	300mg	300 mg
Sodium	Less Than	2,400mg	2,400mg
Total Carbohydrate		300g	375g
Dietary Fiber		25g	30g

Calories per gram:
Fat 9 • Carbohydrate 4 • Protein 4

Recommendations in the U.S. currently call for a maximum of 2,300 milligrams of sodium per day. However, this is reduced to 1,500 milligrams per day if you have hypertension, diabetes, kidney disease, are African-American, or are over 40 (the latter two groups are considered strong risks for developing hypertension). Since almost 70% of Americans fit into one of the aforementioned categories, we should all just shoot for 1,500 milligrams of sodium per day. It can be a bit tedious to add up all of these numbers, but here are some tips that will help you reduce the amount of sodium that you are consuming:

1) Don't add salt to your food at the table. In fact, don't even keep a salt shaker on your table. Human taste buds can't even detect a 25% decrease in a food's sodium level, so chances are you won't even notice the difference.

2) Seventy-five percent of our sodium consumption comes from processed foods (2). Try to eat fewer processed foods and more fresh foods like fruits, vegetables, lean proteins, whole grains, and vegetable oils.

3) Here are the top 10 sources of sodium in the American diet. These numbers are based on a combination of both the amount of sodium in the food and the frequency of consumption.

Top Sources of Sodium In The American Diet

Top Sources of Sodium In The American Diet
Breads And Rolls
Cold Cuts And Cured Meat
Pizza
Poultry
Soups
Sandwiches
Cheese
Pasta Dishes
Meat Dishes
Snack Treats

Source: Reference 7

4) Choose low sodium versions of any canned foods you regularly buy, including soups, sauces, and beans. After a very short while, you won't even notice the difference and can save hundreds of milligrams of sodium per serving.

5) Limit fast foods which are a huge source of sodium in our diets.

6) Shoot for foods with less than 300 milligrams of sodium per serving by reading the food labels before you buy them.

7) Salt substitutes like *Mrs. Dash* are great in place of salt. They are a blend of herbs and spices and add flavor without adding sodium.

8) Eat out less. Restaurants generally use much more salt than you would at home. Eat out at restaurants now and again as a special treat, and eat most of your meals at home.

TAKE HOME MESSAGE

1) All of us should try to limit our consumption of sodium. There are benefits both for those with hypertension as well as for those free of hypertension.
2) Salt has been associated with increased blood pressure, increased risk of heart attack, stroke, and osteoporosis, and may increase risk of gastric cancer.
3) Shoot for 1,500 mg of sodium or less each day. Processed foods account for 75% of the sodium in our diets, so eating fresh unprocessed foods is a great way to decrease your sodium consumption.

References

1) Wardlaw, GM. Perspectives In Nutrition 4th Edition 1999 McGraw Hill Boston, MA.

2) Brown IJ, Tzoulaki I, Candeias V, et al. Salt intakes around the world: implications for public health. *International Journal of Epidemiology*. 2009; 38:791-813.

3) Sacks FM, Svetkey LP, Vollmer WM, et al. Effects on blood pressure of reduced dietary sodium and the dietary approaches to stop hypertension diet. *The New England Journal Of Medicine* 2001; 344:3-10.

4) Strazzullo P, D'Elia L, Kandala NB, et al. Salt intake, stroke, and cardiovascular disease: meta-analysis of prospective studies. *British Medical Journal* 2009; 339:b4567.

5) Devine A, Criddle RA, Dick IM, et al. A longitudinal study of the effect of sodium and calcium intakes on regional bone density in postmenopausal women. *The American Journal of Clinical Nutrition*. 1995;62:740-45.

6) Tsugane S, Sasazuki S, Kobayashi M, et al. Salt and salted food intake and subsequent risk of gastric cancer among middle-aged Japanese men and women. *British Journal of Cancer* 2004; 90:128-34.

7) http://www.cdc.gov/vitalsigns/Sodium/

Priority #7
Choose Whole Grains Instead Of Refined Grains And Get Plenty Of Fiber

The human experience with grains has changed dramatically since our evolutionary times. Early on, we ate grains in a highly unrefined state. They were consumed in their whole form, and all was good with the world. In the last couple of hundred years, and most notably in the past 50 years, this has changed and for the worse.

A grain in its natural form consists of 3 parts: 1) *The Bran*—this is the tough outer layer that protects the inside parts of the grain. 2) *The Endosperm*—this is the starchy part of the grain. 3) *The Kernel*—this is the reproductive center of the grain that sits inside the endosperm. Before refrigeration, the storage and preservation of food was a huge problem. Healthy oils inside the germ can turn rancid over time and cause the grain to spoil. To increase the shelf life of grains, the process of milling was developed in the later 19th century.

Milling strips away the bran and germ and breaks up the starchy endosperm into much smaller particles. Milling dramatically increases the shelf life of grain products but does so at a huge price. Almost all of the vitamins and fiber are removed in the milling process and a once healthy food becomes decidedly unhealthy.

In the U.S., most of the grains we consume are refined, and we are paying the price with our health. Whole grains have been associated with a reduction in risk of heart disease, type 2 diabetes, and inflammatory disease. Let's take a look at some of the most important research on whole grains and health.

Whole Grains And Heart Disease

The association between whole grains and risk of coronary heart disease was examined in 75,521 women from the Nurses' Health Study (1). In 10 years of follow-up, there were 761 new cases of heart disease in this cohort. Women consuming the most whole grains (2.5 servings per day) had a 25% lower risk of heart disease when compared to women who consumed the least amount of whole grains (less than one serving per week). For each increased serving of whole grains, heart disease was reduced by 9%. The researchers believed that the protective effect of whole grains was due to their fiber, vitamin E, and folate content as well as their low glycemic index and reduced insulin demand.

Whole Grains And Colon Cancer

The relationship between whole grains and colon cancer was examined in the very large AARP cohort. Over 197,600 women and over 291,900 men aged 50-71 were followed for five years, during which time there were 2,974 new cases of colon cancer (2). Subjects consuming the most whole grains had a 21% lower risk of colon cancer when compared to those consuming the least amount of whole grains. The anti-cancer effect of the whole grains was thought to be due to their high levels of vitamins, minerals, phenols, and phyto-estrogens.

Whole Grains And Type 2 Diabetes

The association between whole grain consumption and risk of type 2 diabetes was examined in the Nurses' Health Study, the Nurses' Health Study II, and the Health Professional Follow-up Study simultaneously. This was an interesting study that compared the effects of brown rice (a whole grain) and white rice (a refined grain) on the incidence of type 2 diabetes. In total, there were 197,000 men and women followed for an average of about 20 years (3). During this time there were 10,507 new cases of type 2 diabetes in these cohorts.

The researchers found that substituting 50 grams of brown rice for 50 grams of white rice each day would reduce the risk of type 2 diabetes by 16%. This is a big number considering that this is just one food. The researchers believed that the difference in risk was due to the lower glycemic load and higher fiber, vitamin, magnesium, and phytoestrogen levels in brown rice compared to white rice.

Whole Grains And Inflammatory Death

The association between whole grain consumption and inflammatory death was examined in 27,312 women from the Iowa Women's Health Study (4). In this investigation, inflammatory death was considered death from infectious disease, diabetes, asthma, emphysema, rheumatoid arthritis, as well as other causes. After 17 years of follow-up, there were 5,552 deaths related to inflammatory conditions in this cohort. Women who consumed 2½ or more servings of whole grains per day had a 34% lower risk of death from inflammatory causes when compared to women who consumed less than ½ serving of whole grains per day. The authors believed the antioxidant capabilities of the whole grains were responsible for the reduction in risk.

Whole Grain Recommendations

As we just learned, whole grains are an important part of any diet. I have my clients shoot for two servings per day. A serving is a half cup of whole grain. Examples of whole grains include: brown rice, oatmeal, quinoa, corn, and wild rice.

A great way to get started eating whole grains is simply to substitute them for refined grains whenever and wherever you can. Here are a few examples:

Substitute:
Brown rice for white rice
Old fashioned oatmeal for sweetened breakfast cereal
Barilla Plus Whole Grain Pasta for regular pasta
Quinoa for cous cous
Corn on the cob for white potatoes

Whole grains are heartier than refined grains, and most people find that they quickly grow to like the taste of them more than their refined counterparts.

Examples Of Foods High In Fiber And Whole Grains

Whole Grains	High In Fiber
Oatmeal	Fruits
Brown Rice	Vegetables
Quinoa	Beans
Corn	Whole Grains
Wild Rice	Nuts and Seeds

Fiber

One of the ways that whole grains protect us from disease is their high fiber content. Fiber is found in many sources, not just in whole grains. Dietary fiber has been the subject of a large body of research and has been independently associated with disease risk reduction. Therefore, it is worthy of its own section.

What Is Fiber?

In a nutshell, fiber is a carbohydrate that cannot be digested. Fiber is present in fruits, vegetables, whole grains, and legumes. There are really two different types of fiber: 1) *Soluble fiber*—dissolves in water. 2) *Insoluble fiber*—does not dissolve in water.

Insoluble fiber consists of the cell walls of plants. It delays the absorption of sugars and dietary fats. Therefore, insoluble fiber helps to minimize the spikes in blood sugar and insulin levels that we learned is so important to our health in Chapter 4. Examples of insoluble fiber are: brown rice, whole grain breakfast cereals, seeds, carrots, tomatoes, and celery.

Soluble fiber dissolves in the intestine, forming a gelatinous mass. This type of fiber traps bile acids and binds them to the stool. Since bile is so rich in cholesterol, this acts to lower serum cholesterol and reduces risk of coronary heart disease. Good sources of soluble fiber include: oatmeal, legumes, nuts, beans, apples, and berries. Let's take a look at some of the relevant literature concerning fiber and chronic disease.

Fiber And Heart Disease

Nurses' Health Study

The association between fiber and risk of heart disease was examined in 68,782 women from the Nurses' Health Study (5). After 10 years of follow-up, there were 591 new cases of heart disease in this cohort. Women consuming the highest level of fiber

(22.9 grams per day) had a 23% lower risk of heart disease when compared to women consuming the lowest amounts of fiber (11.5 grams per day). For every 10 gram increase in daily fiber consumption, there was a 19% reduction in risk of heart disease. Cereal fiber, found in whole grains, seemed to be the driving force behind the results. The researchers theorized that the decreases in risk were due to the fiber's positive influence on LDL cholesterol, total cholesterol, triglycerides, and insulin sensitivity.

Health Professional Follow-up Study

A similar analysis was conducted in 43,757 men from the Health Professional Follow-up Study (6). After six years of follow-up, there were 734 new cases of myocardial infarction in this cohort. Men consuming the most fiber (28.9 grams per day) had a 36% lower risk of heart disease when compared to men consuming the least fiber (12.4 grams per day). Once again, cereal fiber seemed to be the most important source of fiber. The protective mechanism of fiber in this cohort was thought to be due to its positive impact on serum cholesterol and insulin sensitivity.

Fiber And Type 2 Diabetes

The relationship between fiber and risk of type 2 diabetes was examined in 91,249 women from the younger Nurses' Health Study II cohort (7). After eight years of follow-up, there were 741 new cases of type 2 diabetes in this cohort. Women consuming the most cereal fiber (more than 7.3 grams per day) had a 36% lower risk of type 2 diabetes when compared to women consuming the least cereal fiber (less than 3.8 grams per day). The researchers were not sure what it was about cereal fiber that offered protection against type 2 diabetes when fruit and vegetable fiber were not as significant.

Recommendations For Fiber

A good rule of thumb is to shoot for 14 grams of fiber for each 1,000 calories consumed each day. This translates to around 20 grams per day for most women and around 30 grams per day for most men. Make sure you include sources of both soluble and insoluble fiber, as they are both important and have different health effects. Here are some tips to help you include enough fiber in your diet:

1) Shoot for at least five servings of fruits and vegetables each day, more is better. A serving of fruit is considered one medium sized fruit or ½ cup of cut fruit. A serving of vegetables is equal to ½ cup of cooked or raw vegetables and one full cup of salad greens.
2) Shoot for at least two servings of whole grains each day. Good choices include oatmeal, brown rice, quinoa, and corn.
3) Include nuts and legumes like black beans, chick peas, lentils, and hummus in your protein selections as often as possible.

TAKE HOME MESSAGE

1) In recent years we have dramatically shifted our grain consumption from mostly whole grain to mostly refined. We need to get back to the whole grains.
2) Whole grains reduce risk of chronic disease, including: heart disease, colon cancer, and diabetes.
3) Shoot for at least two servings of whole grains each day. Good sources include oatmeal, brown rice, corn, and quinoa.
4) Fiber from other sources has also been shown to reduce risk of disease. Fiber is found in fruits, vegetables, legumes, nuts, as well as whole grains.
5) Women need about 20 grams of fiber each day, and most men need about 30 grams. Since different types of fiber have distinct health effects, try to get your fiber from a variety of sources.

References

1) Liu S, Stampfer MJ, Hu FB, et al. Whole grain consumption and risk of coronary heart disease: results from the Nurses' Health Study. *American Journal of Clinical Nutrition* 1999; 70:412-19.

2) Schatzkin A, Mouw T, Park Y, et al. Dietary fiber and whole grain consumption in relation to colorectal cancer in the NIH-AARP diet and health study. *American Journal of Clinical Nutrition* 2007; 85:1353-60.

3) Sun Q, Spiegelman D, Van Dam RM, et al. White rice, brown rice, and risk of type 2 diabetes in U.S. men and women. *Archives of Internal Medicine* 2010; 170 (11):961-69.

4) Jacobs DR, Andersen LF, Blomhoff R. Whole grain consumption is associated with a reduced risk of noncardiovascular, noncancer death attributed to inflammatory diseases in the Iowa Women's Health Study. *American Journal of Clinical Nutrition* 2007; 85:1606-14.

5) Wolk A, Manson JE, Stampfer MJ, et al. Long term intake of dietary fiber and decreased risk of coronary heart disease among women. *Journal of the American Medical Association* 1999; 281(21): 1998-2004.

6) Rimm EB, Ascherio A, Giovannucci E, et al. Vegetable, fruit, and cereal fiber intake and risk of coronary heart disease among men. *Journal of the American Medical Association* 1996; 275(6):447-51.

7) Schulze MB, Liu S, Rimm EB, et al. Glycemic index, glycemic load, and dietary fiber intake and incidence of type 2 diabetes in younger and middle aged women. *American Journal of Clinical Nutrition* 2004; 80:348-56.

Priority #8
Eat Plenty Of Fruits And Vegetables

We've all heard from the time we were little kids to eat our fruits and vegetables. It turns out that our mothers and grandmothers knew what they were talking about. Too bad we didn't listen. The typical American averages just 3 servings of fruits and vegetables per day. The typical American needs 3 times this amount.

Fruits and vegetables are jam packed with vitamins, minerals, fiber, antioxidants, flavinoids, phenols, and carotenoids. Fruits and vegetables also have a low glycemic load and a low energy density. These characteristics have a powerful effect on our health.

Fruits and vegetables have been shown to have a positive impact on risks of heart disease, stroke, certain cancers, obesity, diabetes, macular degeneration, and hypertension. Let's take at look at some of the more important research on the association between fruits and vegetables and our health.

Fruit/Vegetable Serving Sizes

1 Piece Of Fruit
½ Cup Of Cut Fruit
½ Cup Of Cut Vegetables
1 Cup Of Salad Greens

Heart Disease

The association between fruit and vegetable consumption and risk of heart disease was examined in 84,251 women from the Nurses' Health Study and 42,148 men from the Health Professional Follow-up Study (1). During 14 years of follow-up for the women and eight years of follow-up for the men, there were 2,190 new cases of heart disease. These cases included both non-fatal myocardial infarction and fatal heart disease.

Subjects consuming the most fruits and vegetables (8 or more servings per day) had a 20% lower risk of coronary heart disease when compared to those consuming the least (less than 3 servings per day). Green leafy vegetables and vitamin C containing fruits and vegetables contributed most to the protective effects.

The authors believed that the protection came from the fruits' and vegetables' high content of antioxidants, folate, fiber, vitamins, and minerals like potassium. These substances may work to decrease risk of coronary heart disease by lowering blood pressure and homocysteine levels or by their antioxidant effects. The authors also went out of their way to mention that white potatoes did not have the same protective effects as other fruits and vegetables.

Stroke

The association between fruit and vegetable consumption and risk of ischemic stroke was examined in 75,596 women from the Nurses' Health Study and 38,683 men from the Health Professional Follow-up Study (2). The women were followed for 14 years, and the men were followed for 8 years. During this time, there were 570 strokes. Men and women consuming the most fruits and vegetables (9.5 servings per day) had a 31% lower risk of ischemic stroke when compared to those consuming the fewest fruits and vegetables per day (2.8 servings per day). Each serving of fruits or vegetables reduced risk of ischemic stroke by 6%.

Cruciferous and green leafy vegetables seemed to drive the results more than other fruits and vegetables. About 5 or 6 servings of fruits and vegetables per day seemed to offer the maximum benefit in this cohort. The authors of the study felt that high levels of dietary fiber, potassium, folate, flavinoids, and/or antioxidants were responsible for the protective effects of the fruits and vegetables.

Cancer

Colon Cancer

The association between fruits and vegetables and colorectal adenomas were examined in 34,467 women in the Nurses' Health Study (3). Colorectal adenomas, also known as polyps, are precursors of most colon cancers, and roughly 15% of adenomas will progress to colon cancer. After 18 years of follow-up, there were 1,720 new cases of adenoma in the distal colon and rectum among these women.

Women consuming 7 or more servings of fruits and vegetables each day had a 19% reduced risk of adenoma when compared to women consuming less than or equal to 3 servings per day. The authors felt that fiber, folate, carotenoids, and/or vitamin C could be the substances in the fruits and vegetables responsible for the protective effect. Fiber in particular has been shown to decrease fecal transit time, increase fecal bulk, lower pH, and produce potentially anti-carcinogenic short chain fatty acids in the digestive system. Folate has also been shown to reduce risk of adenoma. It is likely that the protection is offered through multiple mechanisms.

Renal Cancer

The association between fruit and vegetable consumption and risk of renal (kidney) cancer was examined in 88,759 women from the Nurses' Health Study and 47,828 men from the Health Professional Follow-up Study (4). During 20 years of follow-up for the women and 14 years of follow-up for the men, there were 248 new cases of renal cell cancer. Men who consumed ≥6 servings of fruits and vegetables each day had a 55% lower risk of renal cell cancer when compared to men who consumed less than 3 servings of fruits and vegetables each day. There was no association seen in women.

For the men, each additional serving of a fruit or vegetable was associated with a 9% reduced risk of renal cell cancer. The researchers felt that the carotenoids found in fruits and vegetables had much to do with the protective effect. No explanation was offered for why the effect was not seen in women.

Obesity

The association between fruit and vegetable consumption and risk of obesity was examined in 74,063 women from the Nurses' Health Study over 12 years (5). Women with the largest increase in fruit and vegetable consumption had a 24% lower risk of becoming obese compared to women with the largest decrease in fruit and vegetable consumption. These women also had a 28% reduction in risk of major weight gain (greater than 55 pounds). The researchers believed that the high fiber and low energy density of fruits and vegetables were responsible for the reduced risk of weight gain.

Hypertension

The association between fruit and vegetable consumption and risk of hypertension was examined in 41,541 women from the Nurses' Health Study (6). After four years of follow-up, there were 2,526 new cases of hypertension diagnosed in these women. Intakes of both fruits and vegetables were inversely associated with both systolic and diastolic blood pressure. The researchers felt that the fiber and magnesium present in fruits and vegetables had a lot to do with their blood pressure lowering affects.

Diabetes

The association between fruit and vegetable consumption and incidence of type 2 diabetes was examined in 71,346 women in the Nurses' Health Study. In 18 years of follow-up, there were 4,529 new cases of type 2 diabetes in this cohort (7). Here are some of the major findings of this study:

*An increase in 3 servings of fruit per day reduced risk of type 2 diabetes by 18%.

*One serving per day of green leafy vegetables reduced risk of type 2 diabetes by 9%.

*One serving per day of fruit juice increased the risk of type 2 diabetes by 18%.

The protective effects of fruits were thought to be from their low glycemic index, high fiber, and high micronutrient content. The protective effect of green leafy vegetables was thought to be due to their high levels of magnesium. The increased risk associated with fruit juice consumption was thought to be due to its high glycemic index.

Macular Degeneration

The association between fruit and vegetable consumption and risk of age-related maculopathy was examined in 77,562 women from the Nurses' Health Study and 40,866 men from the Health Professional Follow-up Study (8). The women were followed for 18 years, and the men were followed for 12 years. During this time, there were 464 new cases of age-related maculopathy. Those consuming 3 or more fruits per day had a 36% lower risk of neovascular age-related maculopathy compared to those consuming less than 1½ servings of fruit per day. There was no association found for vegetables.

Fruits are high in antioxidants, which protect against retinal damage. Other compounds in fruits that may be responsible for the protective effects include: flavinoids, phenols, fiber, folate, and potassium.

Recommendations For Fruits And Vegetables

As you can see, a diet high in fruits and vegetables protect you from an impressive number of chronic diseases. There are basically just two recommendations when it comes to fruits and vegetables:

1) *Eat more of them!* Currently, the typical American consumes around 3 servings of fruits and vegetables per day. You want to get that up to at least 5 a day, and preferably closer to 8 or 9. One other thing, white potatoes don't count! They have not been

associated with improved health, and in fact, have been associated with an increased risk of diabetes and weight gain. So, what's a serving? A serving is generally a piece of fruit, ½ cup of chopped fruits or vegetables or a full cup of salad greens.

2) *Go For Variety.* Don't just eat the same fruits and vegetables every day. Each fruit and vegetable has a unique combination of vitamins, minerals, and antioxidants. To get the full spectrum of their protective effects, you need to vary them. The more colors the better. Really mix it up by including reds, blues, whites, blacks, purples, yellows, oranges, etc. They all offer you something different. Here's a list of recommended fruits and vegetables. Work as many of these into your dietary rotation as possible.

A few other notes on fruits and vegetables:

-Remember to limit white potatoes due to their high glycemic index.

-Go a little easy on bananas and grapes. Their lower fiber content tends to make them a bit higher glycemic than other fruits.

-Strictly limit fruit juices and vegetable juices. When you juice a fruit or vegetable, you dramatically increase the sugar content while discarding the fiber.

-Strictly limit dried fruit. As you dry a fruit, you increase the sugar while decreasing the fiber.

Vary Fruit And Vegetable Choices

Apples	Green Pepper
Oranges	Red Pepper
Pineapple	Olives
Blueberries	Carrots
Strawberries	Spinach
Raspberries	Lettuce
Melon	Peas
Grapefruit	Lentils
Watermelon	Black Beans
Mango	Pink Beans
Papaya	Chick Peas
Kiwi	Corn
Pear	Mushrooms
Bananas	Sweet Potato
Grapes	Broccoli
Peaches	Cauliflower
Nectarines	Radishes
Tomatoes	Onion
Brussels Sprouts	Kale

TAKE HOME MESSAGE

1) Fruits and vegetables are the best things you can eat to improve your health.
2) They have been associated with a reduced risk of heart disease, stroke, obesity, diabetes, hypertension, and other diseases.
3) Shoot for at least 5 servings of fruits and vegetables per day, more is better.
4) Vary your fruit and vegetable choices since they all have unique combinations of vitamins, minerals, and antioxidants.

References

1) Joshipura KJ, Hu FB, Manson JE, et al. The effect of fruit and vegetable intake on risk for coronary heart disease. *Annals of Internal Medicine* 2001; 134:1106-1114.

2) Joshipura KJ, Ascherio A, Manson JE, et al. Fruit and vegetable intake in relation to risk of ischemic stroke. *Journal of the American Medical Association* 1999; 282:1233-39.

3) Michels KB, Giovannucci E, Chan AT, et al. Fruit and vegetable consumption and colorectal adenomas in the Nurses' Health Study. *Cancer Research* 2006; 66:3942-53.

4) Lee JE, Giovannucci E, Smith-Warner SA, et al. Intake of fruits, vegetables, vitamin A, C, and E, and carotenoids and risk of renal cell cancer. *Cancer Epidemiology Biomarkers and Prevention* 2006; 15:2445-2452.

5) He K, Hu FB, Colditz GA, et al. Changes in intake of fruits and vegetables in relation to risk of obesity and weight gain among middle-aged women. *International Journal of Obesity* 2004; 28:1569-74.

6) Ascherio A, Hennekens C, Willett WC, et al. Prospective study of nutritional factors, blood pressure and hypertension among U.S. women. *Hypertension* 1996; 27:1065-72.

7) Bazzano LA, Joshipura KJ, Li T, et al. Intake of fruit, vegetables, and fruit juices and risk of diabetes in women. *Diabetes Care* 2008; 31:1311-17.

8) Cho E, Seddon JM, Rosner B, et al. Prospective study of intake of fruits, vegetables, vitamins, and carotenoids and risk of age related maculopathy. *Archives of Ophthalmology* 2004: 122:883-892.

Priority #9
Choose Your Protein Carefully

Eating enough protein is of paramount importance to the maintenance of optimal health. Aside from water, protein forms the major portion of a lean human body, just about 16% of body weight.

Some of the major functions of protein include:

1) *The formation of vital body compounds.* Muscles, enzymes, lipoproteins, connective tissue, clotting factors, immune factors, hormones, and the supporting structures inside bones are all made of protein.

2) *Maintain acid base balance.*

3) *Ensure fluid balance.*

4) *Immune function.* Protein contributes vital parts of the cells used by the immune system.

5) *Provides the body with a ready source of energy.* In general, protein contributes less than 5% of the body's total energy need.

6) *Formation of glucose.* With inadequate carbohydrate intake, the body can make glucose, a major cellular fuel, out of protein's amino acids.

Protein And Health

The impact of protein on our health can certainly be confusing at times. The truth of the matter is that protein itself isn't really in question. It is what comes along with it that is often the problem.

For example, protein in the form of whole grains, nuts, beans, legumes, chicken, and fish come in wonderfully healthy packages. Protein in the form of steak, hot dogs, sausage, bacon, and full fat cheese come in decidedly unhealthy packages.

What you get along with your protein is really the question here. Let's take a look at some of the research on dietary protein and health to sort this all out.

Protein And Coronary Heart Disease

The association between protein and coronary heart disease was examined in 84,136 women from the Nurses' Health Study (1). During 26 years of follow-up, there were 2,210 non-fatal myocardial infarctions and 952 deaths from heart disease in this cohort. Here are some of the major findings from this comprehensive study:

*Women consuming red meat 2 times per day had a 29% increased risk of heart disease when compared to women who consumed an average of ½ serving of red meat per day. In this study, red meat also included processed meats.

*When substituting one serving per day of red meat with one serving per day of...

- -fish: risk of heart disease decreased by 24%.
- -poultry: risk of heart disease decreased by 19%.
- -low fat dairy: risk of heart disease decreased by 13%.
- -nuts: risk of heart disease decreased by 30%.

*High fat dairy was also associated with an increased risk of coronary heart disease.

As you can see, the type of protein consumed can have a dramatically different effect on risk of heart disease. Red meat, processed meat, and high fat dairy products tend to increase risk. Nuts, low fat dairy, chicken, and fish tend to decrease risk.

Red meat is thought to be harmful because of its high iron content. Iron has been associated with an increased risk of myocardial infarction. Furthermore, when cooking red meat, carcinogenic heterocyclic amines can form. These may increase risk of colon cancer. Red meat is also a significant source of saturated fat and cholesterol, which have been shown to increase risk of heart disease. Processed meats are usually high in sodium, which can increase risk of heart disease by raising blood pressure. High fat dairy may increase risk of heart disease due to its high saturated fat content.

Protein And Type 2 Diabetes

The association between a diet high in protein and low in carbohydrate and risk of type 2 diabetes was examined in 85,059 women from the Nurses' Health Study (2). After 20 years of follow-up, there were 4,670 new cases of type 2 diabetes in this cohort. This was actually an investigation that I conducted while studying at Harvard. We found that women who most closely followed a diet high in vegetable protein and vegetable fat and lower in carbohydrate reduced their risk of type 2 diabetes by 18%. This is most likely due to the lower glycemic load of the higher protein diet.

Protein And Stroke

The association between dietary protein and risk of intraparenchymal stroke (a type of bleeding stroke) was examined in 85,764 women from the Nurses' Health Study (3). After 14 years of follow-up, there were 74 intraparenchymal hemorrhages. Women who consumed the most animal protein (82 grams per day) had a 68% lower risk of intraparenchymal stroke when compared to women with the lowest intake (43 grams per day). The reason for the protective effect of the animal protein is likely due to the fact that diets low in protein and saturated fat have been shown to increase risk of this type of stroke.

Red Meat And Colon Cancer

Nurses' Health Study

The association between red meat and colon cancer was examined in 88,751 women in the Nurses' Health Study (4). After six years of follow-up, there were 150 new cases of colon cancer in this cohort. Women who ate red meat every day had 2½ times the risk of colon cancer when compared to women who ate red meat less than once per month.

Processed meats like bacon, sausage, pepperoni, and salami were associated with an increased risk of colon cancer. Fish and skinless chicken were shown to decrease the risk of colon cancer in this cohort. The researchers thought that the nitrosamines and carcinogenic metabolites formed when cooking red meat were responsible for the dramatically increased risk of colon cancer in these women.

Health Professional Follow-up Study

The association between red meat and colon cancer was examined in 47,949 men from the Health Professional Follow-up Study (5). After six years of follow-up, there were 205 new cases of colon cancer in this cohort. Men who ate red meat 5 or more times per week had over 3½ times the risk of colon cancer when compared to those consuming red meat less than once per month.

The researchers felt that the increased risk was due to the high iron consumption of the red meat eaters. Iron can generate hydroxyl radicals when consumed in large amounts. Carcinogenic compounds formed during the cooking of red meat may be another mechanism for the increased risk of colon cancer.

Red Meat And Mortality

The association between red meat and mortality from any cause was examined in 37,698 men from the Health Professional Follow-up Study and 83,644 women from the Nurses' Health Study (6). After 28 years of follow up, there were 23,926 deaths in these cohorts. Men and women consuming the most red meat had a 30% higher risk of death when compared to those consuming the least red meat.

Each additional daily serving of processed red meat was associated with a 20% increased risk of death. Each additional daily serving of unprocessed red meat was associated with a 13% increased risk of death. The researchers believed that higher rates of coronary heart disease and cancer among the red meat eaters was the most likely cause for the increased risk of death in these men and women.

Protein And Weight Loss

An interesting study compared the efficacy of four popular weight loss diets: Atkins (low carb, high protein), Ornish (very low fat, very high carb), the Learn Diet (low fat, high carbohydrate) and the Zone (moderate carb, moderate fat). These diets were studied in 311 obese women over 12 months (7). At the end of the 12 months, the Atkins group lost significantly more weight than the other groups.

Atkins: lost 10.3 pounds
The Zone: lost 3.5 pounds
Ornish: lost 4.8 pounds
Learn Diet: lost 5.7 pounds

The authors cited the higher protein content of the Atkins Diet as a potential mechanism for the increased weight loss.

Protein And Osteoporosis

The association between protein and bone fracture was examined in 85,900 women from the Nurses' Health Study (8). After 12 years of follow-up, there were 234 hip fractures and 1,628 forearm fractures in this cohort. Women consuming the highest amount of protein (95 grams per day) had a 22% increased risk of forearm fracture when compared to women with the lowest protein consumption (68 grams per day). Hip fracture was not associated with protein consumption. The researchers believed that a higher protein diet increased the need for calcium, which is used to buffer the acids that form when digesting high amounts of protein. Calcium can be taken from bone in order to perform this function.

Protein Recommendations

As you can see, protein is quite an interesting macronutrient. If chosen wisely, it can decrease the risk of heart disease, diabetes, and certain kinds of strokes. If chosen poorly, it can increase risk of heart disease and colon cancer. When it replaces refined carbohydrate in the diet, it can help you lose weight. However, consuming too much protein may increase the risk of fracture due to osteoporosis.

Here are some general guidelines on dietary protein:

1) *Pick lean sources of protein that are low in saturated fat*. Here is a list of healthy protein choices:

Healthy Protein Choices

Chicken w/o skin	Monkfish
Turkey w/o skin	Flounder
Low Fat Dairy Products	Tuna (chunk light)
Shrimp	Eggs
Lobster	Black Beans
Crab	Pink Beans
Scallops	Navy Beans
Clams	Chick Peas
Mussels	Lentils
Salmon	Kidney Beans
Scrod	Other Beans
Chilean Sea Bass	Hummus

Here are a few other tips regarding these healthy choices of proteins:

- Limit egg yolks to 6 per week. Eggs are a great food. The yolks, although often criticized, actually provide a lot of vitamins, minerals, and other nutrients. In reality, they are very much like a multivitamin pill. Consuming up to 6 yolks per week has been shown to be safe in the research literature. However, due to their high cholesterol content, you don't want to go overboard with egg yolks, so don't go higher than that. If you have diabetes, it is a good idea to strictly limit egg yolk consumption. Some research has shown an increased risk of heart disease in diabetics who consumed a lot of egg yolks.

-Don't go too overboard with the dairy products. Dairy is a source of protein that is a bit unnatural for humans. We are the only animal to drink another animal's milk, and we are the only animal to drink milk after the age of six months to a year. Remember that milk was designed for an animal with four stomachs. Most people don't digest it very well as they get older. Having said all this, low fat dairy is an excellent source of calcium, which is an important mineral for bone health. I'd say have about 5 servings of low fat dairy per week, but not much more than that.

- Shoot for seafood 3-4 times per week, but not much more than that. Seafood is our best source of omega 3 fatty acids. However, good sources of marine omega 3's are often good sources of mercury. Mercury is a toxic metal that accumulates in predatory fish and can cause neurological problems in adults, children, and developing fetuses. To keep mercury levels low, avoid the biggest sources: tilefish, swordfish, shark, albacore tuna, and king mackerel. Also, keep total seafood intake to 3-4 times per week. If you are pregnant or trying to become pregnant, talk to your doctor about the amount of seafood you should include in your diet.

2) *Avoid sources of protein that are high in saturated fat or are processed red meat.* Here is a list of proteins you should limit. Aim for a maximum of 1 serving per week of lean red meat like filet mignon, pork tenderloin or lean ground beef. Processed red meats like bacon, hot dogs, pepperoni, salami, and other fatty deli meats are particularly harmful. Be sure to strictly limit these foods.

Limit These Sources Of Protein

Whole Milk	Pastrami
Whole Cottage Cheese	Bologna
Whole Yogurt	Sausage
Whole Cheese	Hot Dogs
Hamburger	Bacon
Steak	Other Fatty Cold Cuts
Salami	
Pepperoni	Pork Products

3) *Eat plenty of protein at each meal.* You don't have to limit the amount. Your body won't let you eat more than 20-25% of your calories as protein because it is very high in nitrogen, which is difficult to process. Eating this amount of protein is safe. It will also decrease hunger, make it easier to lose weight, and help to lower the glycemic load of your diet if the protein replaces refined carbohydrates.

4) *Don't go completely overboard with protein and force yourself to eat too much.* There is some evidence that an overabundance of protein may have a negative impact on bone health. If you eat until you're full and not more than this, you'll be fine.

TAKE HOME MESSAGE

1) Dietary protein can be health promoting or damaging to our health, depending on what comes along with it.
2) Lean sources of protein can reduce risk of coronary heart disease, while fatty and processed sources can increase risk.
3) A diet higher in protein and lower in refined grains may help reduce risk of type 2 diabetes and make it easier to lose weight.
4) Eating too much red and processed meat may increase risk of colon cancer.
5) Eating too much protein may have a negative impact on bone health
6) Eat most of your proteins from the "Healthy Protein" list in this chapter and limit choices from the "Less Healthy" list.

References

1) Bernstein AM, Sun Q, Hu FB, et al. Major dietary protein sources and risk of coronary heart disease in women. *Circulation* 2010; 122:876-883.

2) Halton TL, Liu S, Manson JE, et al. Low carbohydrate diet score and risk of type 2 diabetes in women. *American Journal of Clinical Nutrition* 2008; 87:339-46.

3) Iso H, Stampfer MJ, Manson JE, et al. Prospective study of fat and protein intake and risk of intraparenchymal hemorrhage in women. *Circulation* 2001; 103:856-63.

4) Willett WC, Stampfer MJ, Colditz GA, et al. Relation of meat, fat, and fiber intake to the risk of colon cancer in a prospective study among women. *New England Journal of Medicine* 1990; 323:1664-72.

5) Giovannucci E, Rimm EB, Stampfer MJ, et al. Intake of fat, meat, and fiber in relation to risk of colon cancer in men. *Cancer Research* 1994; 54:2390-97.

6) Pan A, Sun Q, Bernstein AM, et al. Red meat consumption and mortality. *Archives of Internal Medicine* 2012; 172(7):555-563.

7) Gardner CD, Kiazand A, Alhassan S, et al. Comparison of the Atkins, Zone, Ornish, and Learn Diets for change in weight and related risk factors among overweight premenopausal women. *Journal of the American Medical Association* 2007; 297:969-977.

8) Feskanich D, Willett WC, Stampfer, et al. Protein consumption and bone fractures in women. *American Journal of Epidemiology* 1996; 143:472-79.

Priority #10
Get Enough Sleep

Many of us feel that getting enough sleep is a luxury and not really a health issue. If you are one of those people, this chapter may really surprise you. Sleep has a major impact on our health, and we simply are not getting enough of it.

According to a recent National Health Interview Survey, nearly 30% of U.S. adults reported an average of less than 6 hours of sleep each night (1). In another study known as the Behavioral Risk Factor Surveillance System, over 35% of respondents reported less than 7 hours of sleep per day in 2009 (2).

Although a lot of what happens when we sleep and why we need so much of it remains something of a mystery, the research is really beginning to mount on the negative health effects of sleep deprivation. Let's take a look at a sample of the research in detail.

Diseases Associated With Sleep Deprivation

Coronary Heart Disease
Type 2 Diabetes
Hypertension
Overweight and Obesity
Early Death

Sleep And Coronary Heart Disease

The association between sleep and coronary heart disease was examined in 71,617 women from the Nurses' Health Study (3). After 10 years of follow-up, there were 934 new cases of heart disease in this cohort. Compared to women getting 8 hours of sleep, those averaging 5 hours or less had a 45% increased risk of heart disease. A surprising finding of this study was that women getting more than 9 hours of sleep had a 38% increased risk of heart disease when compared to women getting 8 hours of sleep.

The authors believed that a lack of sleep increases the risk of heart disease by over-stimulating the sympathetic nervous system. This increases blood pressure and can decrease glucose tolerance. These two conditions increase risk of heart disease. The authors had no explanation as to why getting too much sleep increased the risk of heart disease in this cohort.

Sleep And Type 2 Diabetes

The association between sleep and risk of type 2 diabetes was examined in 70,026 women from the

Nurses' Health Study (4). After 10 years of follow-up, there were 1,969 new cases of type 2 diabetes in this cohort. Women getting less than 5 hours of sleep each night had a 34% increased risk of symptomatic diabetes (a more severe form of diabetes) compared to women getting 8 hours of sleep. Interestingly, women getting 9 or more hours of sleep each night had a 35% greater risk of symptomatic diabetes when compared to women getting 8 hours.

The researchers believed that the increased risk of type 2 diabetes with less sleep was due to impaired glucose tolerance and a decreased insulin sensitivity. The researchers were not sure why too much sleep increased risk in this cohort.

Sleep And Obesity

The association between sleep and weight gain was examined in 68,183 women from the Nurses' Health Study (5). The women were followed for 16 years. Women who slept for 5 hours per night had a 32% increased risk of gaining 15 kilograms (33 lbs.) when compared to women sleeping 7 hours per night. Women only sleeping 6 hours per night had a 12% increased risk of gaining 15 kilograms.

There are a variety of theories as to why a lack of sleep increases weight gain. Sleep deprivation tends to lower leptin levels (a hormone that dictates metabolism) and raise ghrelin levels (a hormone that dictates appetite). The researchers also hypothesized that a decreased thermogenesis may contribute to the weight gain seen in those not getting enough sleep.

Sleep And Blood Pressure

The association between sleep and blood pressure was examined in a randomized trial conducted in Japan (6). Eighteen men between the ages of 23-48 had their blood pressure monitored continuously under 2 conditions: first after a normal 8 hour night of sleep and then after 3.5 hours of sleep. With sleep deprivation, systolic blood pressure rose an average of 6 mm/hg and diastolic blood pressure rose an average of 3 mm/hg. Heart rate also increased by 5 beats per minute after sleep deprivation. The researchers had no explanation as to why these effects occurred with sleep deprivation.

Sleep And Mortality

The association between sleep and death from any cause was examined in 6,928 adults from the Human Population Survey in California (7). Subjects were followed for nine years. Mortality rates for ischemic heart disease, cancer, stroke and all causes combined were lowest for individuals sleeping 7 or 8 hours each night. In fact, men and women sleeping less than 6 hours per night or more than 9 hours per night had a 30% increased risk of dying compared to those sleeping 7 or 8 hours. The authors were unsure of the mechanisms behind the increased risk of death with too little or too much sleep.

Sleep Recommendations

As we've just learned, there is a great deal of evidence that sleep deprivation is harmful to our health. Shoot for at least 7 hours of sleep each night. People who consistently get less than this do so for one of two reasons: 1) They are too busy and their schedule prevents them from getting enough sleep. 2) They can't sleep because either their body or their mind keeps them from falling or staying asleep. We'll look at each of these scenarios one at a time. I have focused on sleep habits quite a bit with my weight loss clients lately since new research shows how important it is to help one lose weight and keep it off.

If You Are Too Busy To Sleep

1) *Make sleep a priority.* It sounds simple enough, but the first strategy is to mentally realize just how important it is to get enough sleep. Look at it as a health issue and something that is not negotiable.

2) *Arrange your schedule so you always get your sleep.* Step 1 is to figure out what time you need to get up in the morning. Step 2 is to subtract 7 hours from then and you've got your new bed time. No matter what is going on, wrap it up at this time and hit the sack.

If you are doing work or studying, stop it and go to bed. Finish up in the morning. If you are watching a great football game or a TV show, turn it off and get to bed. Tivo the rest of it and watch it the next day. Do your best to go to sleep the same time each night and to wake up the same time each morning. This may not always happen on the weekend, but make sure you are tight with this from Sunday through Thursday night.

If You Can't Fall Asleep Or Stay Asleep

1) *Get in the habit of meditation.* If you can't sleep because your mind or body is wired, meditation is almost always the answer. If you get into the habit of doing some type of meditation for 10 minutes or so each night before you go to bed, I guarantee that you will fall asleep quicker and stay asleep with more ease.

You will also notice that you handle stress much better during the day. A really good, simple introduction to meditation is *The Relaxation Response* by Dr. Herbert Benson. Pick this book up! It's a quick read and will help improve the quality of your sleep for the rest of your life.

When you first start, you're going to feel like nothing is happening. After about a month to six weeks, you'll start seeing the benefits. If you find it hard to meditate on your own, pick up a relaxation CD that focuses on deep breathing, muscle relaxation, and/or guided imagery. This works just as well.

2) *White noise.* Sometimes outside noise can wake you up and keep you from sleeping. This can be especially true if you live in a city. Some white noise can drown out these disruptions. I use an air purifier that cleans the air of allergens and provides some gentle white noise. It helps quite a bit.

3) *Go easy on the fluids in the evening.* Many of my clients who can't sleep through the night wake up to use the bathroom and then can't fall back asleep. Limiting coffee and other beverages after 8:00 PM should help to minimize the late night bathroom trips.

4) *Make your bedroom very dark.* For some people, early morning sunlight creeps in and wakes them up. Keep your room really dark to avoid this scenario. You can do this by having really good blinds or pick up a sleep mask to make it 100% dark no matter what time you are sleeping.

5) *Limit late night exercise.* Some people get a bit wired if they do a lot of physical activity shortly before bedtime. A few years back, I was in a hockey league that played their games very late, sometimes starting at 10:00 PM. When I got home and tried to sleep, my body was not close to being ready. Limit cardio several hours before bedtime if you find this to be a problem.

6) *Limit caffeine late at night.* This is probably an obvious one for most, but limiting post dinner caffeinated beverages is a good idea if you are having trouble sleeping.

7) *Increase your physical activity.* While late night exercise can make it hard to sleep, increasing exercise earlier in the day improves sleep dramatically.

8) *Go easy on the alcohol.* Alcohol has been shown to disrupt sleep quality, so cutting back a bit can have a significant impact on your sleep.

9) *Naps count.* If you get less than 7 hours of sleep, you can make up the time with a nap. This may not be possible for everyone, but if you can take advantage of it, you should do so. I recommend a maximum of 30 minutes of nap time. Longer than this can leave you groggy and disrupt the following night's sleep. Therefore, be sure to set an alarm when napping.

TAKE HOME MESSAGE

1) Understand that getting enough sleep is not a luxury but a serious health issue.
2) Getting too little sleep has been associated with an increased risk of heart disease, symptomatic diabetes, obesity, hypertension, and all cause mortality.
3) Shoot for a minimum of 7 hours of sleep each night.

References

1) Schoenborn CA, Adams PF. Health behaviors of adults: U.S. 2005-2007, National Center For Health Statistics *Vital and Health Statistics 10* 2010 245 1-132.

2) http://www.cdc.gov/features/dssleep/

3) Ayas NT, White DP, Manson JE, et al. A prospective study of sleep duration and coronary heart disease in women. *Archives of Internal Medicine* 2003; 163(2):205-209.

4) Ayas NT, White DP, Al-Delaimy WK, et al. A prospective study of self-reported sleep duration and incident diabetes in women. *Diabetes Care* 2003: 26:380-84.

5) Patel SR, Malhotra A, White DP, et al. Association between reduced sleep and weight gain in women. *American Journal of Epidemiology* 2006; 164:947-54.

6) Tochikubo O, Ikeda A, Miyajima E, et al. Effects of insufficient sleep on blood pressure monitored by a new multibiomedical recorder. *Hypertension* 1996; 27:1318-24.

7) Wingard DL, Berkman LF. Mortality risk associated with sleeping patterns among adults. *Sleep* 1983; 6:102-07.

In Conclusion

Now that you've finished reading the book, it is my sincere hope that you understand how much of a role you have in the maintenance of your health. The risks of the top killers in America today are highly modifiable. Of course, it is entirely up to you how you want to deal with this information. I certainly hope that you will be proactive in reducing your risk of chronic disease.

Perhaps you are one of the rare group of people that are already following these recommendations perfectly. If so, good for you, and keep going. If not, try to work on the areas where you are falling short. Every little bit counts, and you are never too old to improve your quality of life and length of days. Remember, the lifestyle habits are listed in order of importance, so make sure that you prioritize your health behaviors accordingly. Let's take one more look at them all at once:

1) Don't Smoke: If you smoke, quit. If you don't, do not start. This is the single most important thing you can do to improve your health.

2) Maintain A Healthy Weight: Second only to smoking is getting your body mass index into a healthy range. Shoot for a BMI of 25 or less.

3) Be Physically Active: To improve your health and limit risk of chronic disease, shoot for 150-180 minutes of cardiovascular exercise each week. If your goal is weight loss, it's more like 250 minutes per week. Also make sure to include some resistance training at least twice per week.

4) Choose Low Glycemic Load Sources Of Carbohydrate: Strictly limit refined carbohydrates like white bread, pasta, white rice, and sugar. Instead, focus on fruits, vegetables, beans, and whole grains like oatmeal, brown rice, and quinoa.

5) Choose Your Fats Carefully: Strictly limit saturated fat and totally avoid trans fat. Focus on poly- and monounsaturated fats like nuts, seeds, vegetable oil, nut butters, and avocados. Remember, low fat isn't the way to go either, shoot for 30-35% of your calories as healthy fats.

6) Limit Sodium: Shoot for no more than 1500 mg of sodium per day.

7) Eat Some Whole Grains Each Day And Be Sure To Get Plenty Of Fiber: Make sure to include whole grains like oatmeal, brown rice, and quinoa on a regular basis and get lots of fiber from other sources like fruits, vegetables, and beans.

8) Eat Plenty Of Fruits And Vegetables: Get at least 5 servings of fruits and vegetables each day, even more is better.

9) Choose Your Protein Carefully: Limit red meat and processed meats like steak, bacon, sausage, and pork and focus on healthy sources of protein like beans, nuts, whole grains, chicken, turkey, and fish.

10) Get Enough Sleep: Sleep is the foundation of our health. Get at least 7 hours per night.

If you are able to heed these recommendations, I am more than convinced that you will dramatically reduce your risk of chronic disease. Incidentally, you will greatly increase the quality of your life at the same time. These recommendations will improve your physique, give you more energy, boost your immune system so you'll get sick less, reduce the effects of stress on your body, help fight anxiety and depression, boost your self confidence, and even improve your sex life. You'll get a lot back for focusing on these 10 lifestyle habits.

As we've seen throughout this book, these factors taken individually have a dramatic impact on your health. But what happens when you combine them? Harvard sought to answer this question with a study it published in the prestigious *New England Journal of Medicine* (1). The article was titled: *Primary prevention of coronary heart disease through diet and lifestyle.*

The outcome in this study was coronary heart disease, the number one killer in the U.S. The researchers created a scoring system for each of the 84,129 women from the Nurses' Health Study that were included in the investigation. The scoring was calculated as follows:

1) *Smoking Status:* Women who were not currently smoking received a score of "1", women who were currently smoking received a score of "0".

2) *Weight:* Women who had a body mass index under 25 received a score of "1", if their body mass index was 25 or higher, they received a score of "0".

3) *Alcohol:* Women who consumed an average of ½ drink of alcohol per day received a score of "1", if not they received a score of "0" (moderate alcohol consumption has been associated with a reduced risk of coronary heart disease).

4) *Physical Activity:* Women who engaged in moderate to vigorous physical activity (including brisk walking) for 30 minutes or more per day received a score of “1”, women who did not received a score of “0”.

5) *Diet:* A composite dietary score was also created. To receive a score of 1, women needed to be in the top 40% of a diet:

1) High in cereal fiber, marine omega-3 fatty acids, folate, and ratio of polyunsaturated fat to saturated fat.

2) Low in trans fat and dietary glycemic load.

If not they received a score of “0”.

During 14 years of follow-up there were 1,128 new cases of coronary heart disease. Women who scored a perfect 5 out of 5 had an 83% lower risk of coronary heart disease. The population attributable risk was 82%. This means that 82% of the coronary events in this cohort might have been prevented if all of the women in the cohort had practiced these lifestyle habits.

83% Lower Risk of Heart Disease In Women In The Nurses' Health Study If They....

Did Not Smoke Maintained A Healthy Weight Consumed Moderate Amounts of Alcohol Exercised 30 Minutes Per Day Consumed A Healthy Diet

Source: Reference 1

If you were to generalize this to the entire country, potentially 82% of all heart disease events would be avoided if everyone did all five of these things. That's more than 8 out of 10 coronary events avoided! Keep in mind that heart disease is the number one killer in this country, and this study shows that when you take good care of yourself, it is extremely preventable. This investigation is a great example of how the combination of these lifestyle factors can dramatically reduce the risk of chronic disease. This is powerful stuff.

The one problem with the study is that only 3% of the cohort had a perfect score of 5! I'm sure that this number is even lower for the country as a whole. We clearly have a lot of work to do.

Hopefully, you will agree that I have met my goals in writing this book. It was my goal for each reader to:

1) Understand that much of their health is in their own hands. Not all of it, but much more than most people think.

2) Learn a bit about the research on lifestyle and health. There is a huge body of well designed research out there that has much to teach us, and most people don't know that it exists or how to interpret it.

3) Evaluate your current lifestyle and identify the areas where you are doing well and those areas where you need some work.

4) Lastly, it is my sincere hope that you will take the necessary steps to work on any areas where you need improvement. This will lead you to greater health, longevity, quality of life, and allow you to reach your potential as a human being.

Here's to your good health!

Dr. Thomas L. Halton

References

1) Stampfer MJ, Hu FB, Manson JE, et al. Primary prevention of coronary heart disease in women through diet and lifestyle. *New England Journal of Medicine* 2000; 343:16-22.

Also By Dr. Thomas L. Halton:

The Weight Loss Triad
A Comprehensive Guide To Lasting Weight Loss

Life On The Triad
Meal Plan And Recipe Companion For *The Weight Loss Triad*

19406039R00087

Made in the USA
Lexington, KY
17 December 2012